Praise for *Brain Fitness*

"*Brain Fitness*, written by Dr. Aihan Kuhn, is a remarkable book. In this guide, Dr. Kuhn offers clear, concise explanations of how our brains work and how we can optimize our mental processing through qigong and tai chi. Her premise that brain aging can be prevented through body movement is well founded and has been demonstrated by modern neuroscience. By following the specific exercises that Dr. Kuhn prescribes in *Brain Fitness*, the reader will be able to think, work, and live productively with an enhanced sense of clarity and calm."

—Catherine Kurosu, MD, LAc.

"I am amazed at Dr. Aihan Kuhn's ability to explain the principles, benefits, and practices of the ancient Chinese exercises tai chi and qigong, seemingly incomprehensible to the public, in such an easy-to-understand way. If you want to improve energy and blood flow in your body, enhance your immune function, improve your daily energy level and mental sharpness, and delay your aging process, *Brain Fitness* will teach you how to meet your goals."

—Shi-Fa Ding, PhD; senior scientist,
SQI Diagnostics, Inc., Toronto, Canada

"A guide offers exercises for the mind, body, and spirit.

"Mixing Western medicine with Eastern traditions, Kuhn . . . introduces the reader to two worthy 'internal energy workouts': taiji and qigong. Both blend meditation and exercise and are, according to the author, excellent ways to counter the damages of aging that affect bodies and minds. Taking a holistic approach to health, Kuhn advocates a regimen of simple exercises that will keep the body in balance, sharpening memory and holding diseases at bay: 'If you move your body in an energetic way every day,' writes Kuhn, 'you can change your life and your health.' Following an explanation of the history and philosophy of qigong and its younger offshoot, taiji, the author describes the positive effects of these practices on the cardiovascular, respiratory, gastrointestinal, and nervous systems, as well as how they increase stamina, bolster the immune system, and correct chemical imbalances. She then goes through the various exercises, providing photographic examples and paragraphs explaining the goals and payoffs of each one. The author also advises the reader on other activities—such as singing and socializing—that supplement these exercises. Excerpts from the *Tao Te Ching* and a list of recommended reading round out this primer for anyone embracing these Chinese workouts. Kuhn writes in a clear prose that is simple to follow. She makes a compelling case for the exercises and the philosophy behind them. Even those who are unconvinced of the validity of traditional Chinese medicine should find sound advice for healthy living in these pages. But some chapters feel redundant, repeating information—such as the benefits of taiji—found elsewhere in the book. Similarly, a vague mystical language permeates the volume ('Shen refers to our spiritual energy, our highest consciousness, a reconnection with universal energies'), which may put off more skeptical readers. But those curious about traditional Chinese exercise or interested in a holistic program of health with a philosophical bent should find much of value in this work. As Kuhn likes to remind the reader, these are exercises for all ages, and the younger one starts, the better.

"An informative manual for explorers of taiji and qigong."

—*Kirkus Reviews*

BRAIN FITNESS

The Easy Way of
Keeping Your Mind Sharp
Through Qigong Movements

Dr. Aihan Kuhn
CMD, OBT

Also by Dr. Aihan Kuhn

Natural Healing with Qigong
Simple Chinese Medicine
Tai Chi for Depression
Tai Chi in 10 Weeks

BRAIN FITNESS

The Easy Way of Keeping Your Mind Sharp Through Qigong Movements

Dr. Aihan Kuhn
CMD, OBT

YMAA Publication Center
Wolfeboro, NH USA

YMAA Publication Center, Inc.
PO Box 480
Wolfeboro, New Hampshire 03894
1-800-669-8892 • info@ymaa.com • www.ymaa.com

ISBN: 9781594395246 (print) • ISBN: 9781594395253 (ebook)

Edited by Leslie Takao and Doran Hunter
Cover design by Axie Breen
Photos by YMAA unless noted
This book is typeset in Minion Pro and Fairfield LT Std

Names: Kuhn, Aihan, author.
Title: Brain fitness : the easy way of keeping your mind sharp through qigong movements /
    Dr. Aihan Kuhn.
Description: Wolfeboro, NH USA : YMAA Publication Center, [2017] | Includes bibliographical
    references and index.
Identifiers: ISBN: 9781594395246 (print) | 9781594395253 (ebook) | LCCN: 2017940328
Subjects: LCSH: Qi gong—Health aspects. | Tai chi—Health aspects. | Qi gong—Psychological aspects. |
    Tai chi—Psychological aspects. | Intellect—Deterioration—Prevention. | Memory disorders—
    Prevention. | Brain—Aging—Prevention. | Brain—Degeneration—Prevention. | Holistic medicine. |
    Medicine, Chinese. | Mind and body. | Self-care, Health. | LCGFT: Self-help publications. | BISAC:
    SELF-HELP / Personal Growth / Memory Improvement. | BODY, MIND & SPIRIT / Healing /
    Energy (Qigong, Reiki, Polarity) | HEALTH & FITNESS / Diseases / Alzheimer's & Dementia. |
    SELF-HELP / Aging. | SELF-HELP / Self-Management / Stress Management.
Classification: LCC: RC394.M46 K86 2017 | DDC: 616.8/4—dc23

Disclaimer

This book is intended to assist people concerned about brain aging and memory loss, to help taijiquan students understand the true nature of taiji and qigong practice, and to help them achieve the maximum benefits from learning taiji, especially its antiaging benefits.

The practice, treatments, and methods described in this book should not be used as alternatives to professional medical diagnosis or treatment. The author and publisher of this book are NOT RESPONSIBLE in any manner whatsoever for any injury or negative effects that may occur through following the instructions and advice contained herein.

It is recommended that before beginning any treatment or exercise program you consult your medical professional to determine whether you should undertake this course of practice.

Printed in Canada.

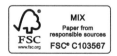

Editorial Notes

Romanization of Chinese Words

The interior of this book primarily uses the Pinyin romanization system of Chinese to English. In some instances, a more popular word may be used as an aid for reader convenience, such as "tai chi" in place of the Pinyin spelling, *taiji*. Pinyin is standard in the People's Republic of China and in several world organizations, including the United Nations. Pinyin, which was introduced in China in the 1950s, replaces the older Wade-Giles and Yale systems.

Some common conversions are found in the following:

Pinyin	Also spelled as	Pronunciation
qi	chi	chē
qigong	chi kung	chē gōng
qin na	chin na	chǐn nǎ
jin	jing	jǐn
gongfu	kung fu	gōng foo
taijiquan	tai chi chuan	tī jē chǔén

For more information, please refer to *The People's Republic of China: Administrative Atlas*, *The Reform of the Chinese Written Language*, or a contemporary manual of style.

Formats and Treatment of Chinese Words

The first instances of foreign words in the text proper are set in italics. Transliterations are provided frequently: for example, Eight Pieces of Brocade (Ba Duan Jin, 八段錦).

Chinese persons' names are mostly presented in their more popular English spelling. Capitalization is according to the *Chicago Manual of Style* 16th edition. The author or publisher may use a specific spelling or capitalization in respect to the living or deceased person. For example: Cheng, Man-ch'ing can be written as Zheng Manqing.

To my husband, Gerry;
my son, Peter; and my daughter, Sharon

Acknowledgments

It took a great deal of time and effort to figure out how to say things right, how to put English-language sentences in the right order and make them communicate the way I wanted them to. In Chinese, we speak and write in the opposite order from English. So we say, "English speaks opposite." On the other hand, English speakers would say *we* speak in the opposite order. I have improved a great deal in my speaking and my writing, but I am learning all the time. To finish this book, I still needed a lot of help. Luckily, I have many very good people around me, giving me support, not only with my language but also with many other aspects of my work and my life. Therefore, I would like to take this opportunity to thank all the people who have helped me, who reviewed this book, who made many corrections, and who gave me a great deal of encouragement.

A taiji book is not too hard for me to write because I have been teaching it for more than twenty years. To clearly describe the benefits to our brains, however, is much more complicated. I've done a lot of research, reading, and studying, trying to identify the connections between Eastern and Western science and to explain why taiji is so beneficial. I would like to thank Marie Murphy and Michele Talabach, who have been teaching young people with learning disabilities and behavior problems and providing counseling at the college level for many years. I would also like to thank Pam Formosa, a longtime Brain Gym teacher. She told me, "There are many similarities between Brain Gym, qigong, and taiji"—words that helped convince me that I was on the right track. I would like to thank my good friend Mary Beth Kahler, who helped me with language issues any time I needed it.

I am very thankful to my husband, Gerry Kuhn, always the first person to read my drafts and do the first round of editing. I would like to thank my son, Peter Kuhn, who has helped me with both my work and my language. I would also like to thank Ron Weinberg, who is always watching over me and helping me on my path to success.

Thanks go as well to our taiji instructors and assistant instructors, Jeanne Donnelly, Joe Foley, Shawn Armacost, Alon Harpaz, and Vic Cevoli. Even though some of them have moved away, their feedback has always helped me in both communicating about taiji and gathering data about its practice.

Thank you to everyone who read and appreciated my first book, *Natural Healing with Qigong* and my second book, *Simple Chinese Medicine*, which has been honored as a finalist in the Health: Alternative Medicine category of the National Best Books 2009 awards, sponsored by *USA Book News*. Thanks especially to those readers who gave me so much positive feedback on Amazon. You gave me the encouragement to continue writing and exploring human energy science, preventive medicine, and natural healing.

I always remind myself I have much to be grateful for, and I am very thankful for all the help I receive.

Dr. Aihan Kuhn

Table of Contents

Preface

I studied conventional Western medicine in medical school in China from 1977 to 1982. Much of the information in this book is based on general information I learned in medical school blended with practical knowledge I gathered from my natural healing practice. The information in this book also comes from other reputable sources. I have done my best to synthesize my taiji experience with my medical and scientific knowledge.

When I was young, I used to wonder why taiji and qigong masters were so smart, so healthy, so calm, and so cool. When I started to learn taiji, I just wanted to be like them. In the first several years, although I didn't come near to their achievements, I did feel good overall, in health and well-being. Now I have been teaching and practicing for a long time, and as the years have gone by, I have started to see the difference. I have begun to see myself as a different person, as a master of my own life.

I used to have a poor memory, perhaps from my poor genes. My parents had poor health. My mother and her family had arthritis, and my father had tuberculosis when he was nine years old. In middle age, he had chronic bronchitis and asthma, which often turned to pneumonia. He also had chronic obstructive pulmonary disease, or COPD. My poor memory showed in school—especially medical school. It took me twice as long to learn, sometimes three times as long as my classmates to memorize the coursework.

In Chinese medicine, the brain is related to kidney energy. If you have poor kidney energy (and I was apparently born this way), you will have memory, arthritis, hair, teeth, and bone issues. Actually, I have all of these. My saving grace is that I am a taiji and qigong practitioner. Even though I have many issues, I don't have too many symptoms that affect my life, work, or career. I attribute this to my practice. Also, my memory—which should be getting worse with age—has not diminished. But it is almost the same as it was when I was young. In some ways, it is even better than before.

My learning ability has improved too. I wasn't born smart. I could never picture myself using a computer before. I used to get lost when driving even though I'd been to my destination before. I had a hard time reading a map. It was just too confusing. I remember one time at night when I finished teaching a class at a new place, I drove thirty miles in the wrong direction while trying to get home. I ended up calling the police department to have a policeman guide me back to the highway. By the time I got home, it was almost midnight. And I would never have thought I could speak in public. I could barely make it through talks with groups of friends when I was younger. Here, living in a different country and struggling with English, it's even worse. How could I ever give public speeches? Now I do use a computer every day, and I often get compliments from my computer-geek husband. I make fewer wrong turns when I go to new places, and I can use a map very well now. I regularly give speeches all over, at trainings, lectures, workshops, and in the course of teaching. I attribute all of these improvements to my taiji and qigong practice and teaching.

I share this with you because I believe anyone who is willing to change and put in the effort for self-improvement will see results. Besides, taiji and qigong simply make you feel good. Who doesn't want to feel good? Taiji is a journey, a healthful journey—a way to a better life.

Dr. Aihan Kuhn

Chapter 1

Body-Brain-Mind Healing

What Matters in Our Lives?

FOR MANY YEARS, I have been focused on treating disease. That is what I was trained to do. All doctors, Eastern and Western, are taught to treat disease, and that's what I always thought medicine was about. Over the past fifteen years, however, I have shifted from treating only disease to treating the whole person. This happened, at least in part, because I was not happy with the health-care system here in the United States. I was not satisfied with doctors who would spend only five to ten minutes with me and then simply give me a prescription without truly understanding what was going on with my health. I expected that doctors would explain to me why I had this problem, how I would be helped, and what I could do to prevent it from recurring. I then started attending conferences, workshops, lectures, and furthering my reading to understand more about the body. I started to integrate everything I had learned from both Eastern and Western medicine and used all this information to help my patients. I found that I grew spiritually, intellectually, and practically in my healing ability as all these viewpoints came together. When my patients' health improved—miraculously, it seemed to me—I was convinced that my strategy and approaches were right.

For the past five years, I have started to focus on some of my own issues, particularly my brain health, so that I can be at my best and get the most enjoyment possible from my life. I need my brain to be healthy for my quality of life, for conducting business, for creating new methods to achieve health and fitness, for teaching, for healing, for helping others, and for fighting my own aging process. It may sound like I'm doing this all for myself, but I am merely the subject of my own experimental research. I wish both to heal myself and to find out if my right-brain dominance can really change. What I discover I can then pass on to others.

After years of practicing taiji and qigong, doing exercises I have created myself, and employing other methods I have learned, I have changed in many ways. I had fear and anger before but no longer. I had anger before, and now it's all gone. I had high expectations for myself and my family. Now I only do the work I love and let others be whoever they want to be. I used to be very stubborn, but now I can let things go much more easily. I used to be overly skeptical, but now I am open to everything. I tended to fight if I thought I was right about something, but now I'd rather enjoy peace. It really doesn't matter who is right and who is not (there is no absolute right and wrong anyway). I used to think I knew everything, but now I know I am still learning every day, and I have so much more to learn. All these experiences and benefits are evidence to me that our minds, bodies, brains, and the ways we heal are interrelated, and all are important.

Many things can cause stress and bring about premature aging. Stress is a great hazard to life, health, healing, and learning. It affects the brain and its functions, like memory. Stress can come from work, home, physical ailments, diet, negative thoughts, politics, financial burdens, lack of support, dealing with unprofessional and irresponsible people, worrying about retirement, relationships, fear, driving and traffic, children, parents, spouse, the news, bills and taxes, the environment, and so many things. Stress causes tension in our bodies, affecting energy flow, which then affects our health from head to toe. We may suffer everything from poor productivity to memory loss, depression, heart disease, stroke, and cancer. Other ailments caused by stress include headaches, insomnia, anxiety, back pain, chest pain, hypertension, poor immune system, indigestion, irritable bowel syndrome, substance abuse, anger, and social withdrawal.

Despite our society's increased focus on stress reduction, the amount of stress has not lessened. And people who teach stress reduction are no less stressed than anyone else. High technology neither relieves our stress nor reduces the tension in our bodies, but it can make us lazy in a way. We get too much information, too much stimulation, and too much negativity, all of which trouble our minds. Our minds are simply too busy. It's no wonder many people forget things. We become distracted and don't pay attention to our feelings, our bodies, and our health. We don't know how to breathe or how to relax, and we become depleted. We are not aware of our own energy, which is so crucial to our well-being.

If we don't start paying attention to ourselves, we'll never be able to understand ourselves. We won't be able to solve our problems and move forward. We cannot heal ourselves if we don't understand ourselves.

More and more, we have the ability to gain this understanding, including in the area of brain health. There has been a great deal of interest in studying the brain as our investigatory tools have improved and our scientific knowledge has continued to increase. In 1993 the journalist Bill Moyers did a program on public television called *Healing and the Mind*. It had a good influence on Americans. Joan Borysenko's *Minding the Body, Mending the Mind*[1] also had a big impact. Many holistically oriented physicians have become widely popular, including Christiane Northrup, Deepak Chopra, Andrew Weil, and Mehmet Oz. Still, despite the wider prevalence of mind-body medicine, Americans continue to have multiple health problems. Something is missing from the picture.

There is no doubt that the mind can affect the body and even heal the body. In my practice, I teach people how to build a strong mind and then use their mind to help with the healing of their body's illnesses. But I have to teach how to use the body to heal the mind as well. In my experience, using the body to heal the mind has proven to work much better than using the mind to heal the body. Sometimes the mind simply cannot heal the body. This can be seen in people who are really stuck and cannot change their mind-set at all. Sometimes the mind just won't bend or be made to go in the right direction. We have to find another way. And that is to use the body to heal the mind. This is what I think has been missing in much of mind-body medicine.

The Body Can Heal the Mind

After many years of working with patients, treating patients, teaching patients, and observing patients, I developed my own theory: Body-Brain-Mind Healing. My idea is to use physical exercises and movement to stimulate the brain and get the brain chemicals activated. By balancing the left and right sides of the brain, upper and lower brain, cross brain, frontal and back brain through body movements and bringing new information to the brain, we help brain cells communicate with each other. An activated and balanced brain can guide the mind in the right direction, directing the physical body toward positive behaviors and activities. Then the healing begins.

1. Joan Borysenko, *Minding the Body, Mending the Mind* (Reading, MA: Addison-Wesley, 1987).

What happens in the complicated human body involves a wholeness that results from many chain reactions. The mind is not the only player. To instigate a chain reaction that begins in the mind and ends in the body, something needs to set it in motion. To get the mind on the right track, something needs to make the mind work better. The mind can be stuck in the past, searching for the reasons why things happened. Stress can make the mind confused, vulnerable, and debilitated. This is not because our minds are bad or weak, nor because we are stupid. It is because the chemicals in our brains are not balanced, and this affects our emotions. When the emotion centers in our brains are not balanced, our minds become unbalanced.

Fortunately, no matter how stuck our minds may be, our bodies can still move. If you are capable of doing normal daily activities, such as housework or driving, you can certainly move your body enough to enjoy the variety of exercises proposed here. If you move your body in an energetic way every day, you can change your life and your health.

I have been quite successful in incorporating taiji, qigong, and other types of body movements into my patient care. Combining and integrating these treatment modalities into a whole package, along with teaching and guiding patients, have brought my health-care practice to a much higher level. The results: healing, learning, and personal development have changed many lives.

Begin Your Journey

In my daily observation of people and after practicing natural health care for more than thirty years, I have noticed one thing that many people cannot overcome, and that is fear. Fear can make you unable to see things from the proper perspective. It stops you from moving forward. It prohibits you from seeing the possibilities and discovering your potential. If you open your mind to possibilities, and you are willing to try many different things, you might find yourself in a different place. There is a vast amount of information available today about health and healing. But you don't know what really works until you try it yourself.

Some people tell me they cannot change the way they live and the way they eat because they were brought up to behave this way. They don't seem to understand that changing is how we move forward. After teaching taiji and qigong for so many years,

I have seen so many students change, including those who said they could not. This shows the power of these ancient exercises and physical movements.

All you need to do is to open your mind to everything, to all that is, and you will open to new possibilities, new opportunities, and a new way of life. It may not be easy at first, but it is very rewarding, especially as the many benefits manifest in later life.

As with so many things, the best way of learning the art of healing and well-being is by experience. To find out how much you can get from taiji practice, start your journey today. I know it will be wonderful.

Chapter 2

Understanding Taiji and Qigong

TAIJIQUAN IS AN ANCIENT Chinese martial arts exercise, well known for its ability to improve physical, spiritual, emotional, and mental health. It is also effective for disease prevention, healing, antiaging, and self-defense. Taiji is a well-rounded and well-balanced form of exercise. The slow, circular movements require concentration and breath control and allow you to move your internal energy, or life force, with your *intention*. The Chinese word for this life force is *qi* (chi). Moving qi empowers your body and calms your mind. We call this "meditation in motion." It has been proven for centuries that taiji practice offers great health benefits, including improvement in circulation, metabolism, flexibility, posture, concentration, immune function, daily energy level, digestion and absorption, emotional balance, self-awareness, relationship health, harmony in your life, and more. Decades of observation and study have shown that taiji offers great benefits to our brains. Taiji is not just for seniors; it is an exercise for all ages, all races, all religions, all men and women. It is a gift from the Chinese culture, and we can all benefit from it, cherish it, and use it to nourish our energy.

Taiji helps prevent brain aging. This is why people who practice taiji over their lifetimes have good overall health. They are multitalented, clear minded, and logical in their thinking and reasoning. They are more creative and aware and are better able to deal with life's challenges.

Qigong (sometimes spelled chi gung or qi gong) is also an ancient Chinese exercise and offers many of the same benefits as taiji. However, qigong is an easier form of internal energy exercise for health, well-being, antiaging, and healing. Qigong is easier to learn and easier to practice than taiji. The beauty of qigong is that you get results sooner. But both of these exercises are part of anti-brain-aging practice. For more information about qigong, see my book *Natural Healing with Qigong* (YMAA, 2004).

What Is Taiji?

Taiji is the abridged name of taijiquan. "Tai" in Chinese means "bigger than big," "ji" means "extreme," while "quan" means "boxing." Altogether, taijiquan can be translated as "grand force boxing." Taiji's focus is on inner energy and achieving inner peace through movement, although taiji certainly has its martial aspect. In the United States, most people just say *taiji* and skip the *quan*. It is easier to say, and most of us use it for health anyway, not for fighting.

Taiji is an *art,* a beautiful art of *motion.* Performing taiji is like dancing in the clouds. That is why it intrigues people from all over the world. It is lovely both to watch and to experience internally. This is why you get pleasure from within yourself as well as from seeing others practice. I call this kind of pleasure a natural tranquilizer. Unlike other tranquilizers, however, taiji is no depressant.

Taiji is also a form of *meditation,* sometimes called walking meditation or moving meditation, as I mentioned above. This kind of meditation helps you to focus on the present moment, on your own energy center. You can simply detach yourself from old, disturbing memories. It helps you to relieve stress, untangle your troubled life, and get rid of much of the junk that might be interfering with your happiness.

Taiji is an *energy workout* that builds your strength both internally and externally. Qigong is also thought of as an energy workout, and taiji is considered its highest level. These kinds of energy practice can improve energy and blood flow in your body, enhance your immune function, and improve your daily energy level and mental sharpness.

Taiji is a *training involving discipline and focus.* This type of training and discipline can help you improve many things in your life and help you reach your future goals. But developing this discipline and getting the most benefit from taiji requires daily practice, not just practicing occasionally.

Taiji is a *martial art,* derived from the whole body of martial arts. In every movement of taiji, you can find a martial application that can be used for self-defense. As your practice proceeds to higher levels and you continue to study taiji in depth, you will notice this more and develop these self-defense skills.

Taiji is *preventive medicine*—energy medicine or natural healing medicine—because it enhances your self-healing ability, balances your energy, and prevents disease.

For people who have chronic ailments where conventional medicine offers no relief, taiji can assist healing. For people who have cancer, taiji is an excellent natural medicine that enhances the immune system. Taiji is also a social medicine. Because it teaches us to focus on ourselves and strengthen our own energy, it prevents violence and other social problems.

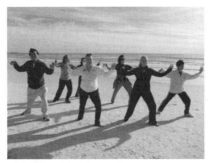

Photo provided by author

Mind-Body-Spirit

Learning and practicing taiji and qigong is a wonderful lifestyle. People from all over the world practice taiji and qigong for the benefits they offer to the mind, the body, and the spirit. Taiji is a mind-body-spirit exercise, whereas most Western-style exercises are mainly focused on developing the body.

The *mind* is the thinking part of our existence responsible for our ability to read, analyze data, use computers, solve problems, and make plans. The *body* is the physical part of our existence: eating, sleeping, walking, jogging, cooking, and other physiological functions. And the *spirit* is the meaningful part of our existence; this is where our hopes, our dreams, fears, love, and hate are expressed. All of these are equally important. Taiji has the potential to bridge these separate parts by putting the practitioner in a state of mind where the connections among them are clear. While taiji exercises the body directly, it has subtle effects on body chemistry in general and on brain chemistry in particular, thus affecting mood and indirectly affecting the spirit. It requires concentration and attention to detail while being practiced, so we are literally exercising the mind as well.

Taiji touches all aspects of the whole person at the same time, reinforcing the notion that these so-called separate parts are but different aspects of the same concept. Taiji helps open the body's energy pathways when practiced through mind, body, and spirit. It is not enough to simply copy the physical movements. You must incorporate them with the other parts of yourself through relaxation, concentration, study of ancient texts, meditation, and dedication to your practice.

Jing, Qi, Shen

In Chinese medicine, there are three fundamental substances called *jing*, *qi*, and *shen*. They in some way refer to our Western terms *body*, *mind*, and *spirit* and work side by side to keep us healthy.

Jing refers to a fundamental substance in the body stored in the kidney. Jing is usually translated as *essence* and has a very close relationship to the Western term *gene* or *genetic material*. It is crucial to the development of the individual throughout life. It is inherited at birth and allows us to develop from childhood to adulthood and then into old age. It governs growth, reproduction, and development; promotes kidney qi; and works with qi to help protect the body from external pathogens. Any developmental disorder such as learning difficulties and physical disabilities in children may be due to a deficiency of jing from birth. Other disorders such as infertility, poor memory, a tendency to get sick or catch colds, and allergies may also be due to deficiency of jing.

Qi refers to vital energy or life-force flow in the body, like the electric flow in a wire. There are various types of qi in the body working together to keep our physical atmosphere in harmony. Qi has a very close relationship to human metabolism, immune function, digestion, absorption, emotion, breathing, mental clarity, and more. Qi is present internally and externally and controls the function of all parts of the body. Qi is the motor of the body, just like the motor in the car. Qi keeps us moving and functioning, keeps us warm, and protects us against sickness. Everything we do involves qi. Walking, eating, laughing, crying, playing sports, working, hiking, and writing are all related to qi. Qi affects our lives every day. We cannot see the qi in the body, but we can feel it. We can feel when our energy is low and when it is high. We can sense if we are optimistic or depressed; we can feel if our bodies are out of balance. Qi is very important in the body and in life.

Shen refers to our spiritual energy, our highest consciousness, a reconnection with universal energies.

The English word *spirit* has many differing meanings and connotations but commonly refers to a supernatural being or essence, transcendent and therefore metaphysical in its nature. The *Concise Oxford Dictionary* defines it as "the non-physical part of a person." For many people, however, spirit, like soul, forms a natural part of a being, not a transcendence of some sort. Such people may identify spirit with mind or with consciousness or with the brain.

Some people refer to shen as a soul. In Chinese medicine theory, shen and soul are two different concepts with some similarities. Soul is the immaterial or eternal part of a living being, commonly held to be *separable in existence* from the body. Shen in traditional Chinese medicine (TCM) is the higher or *energized eternal* part of a living being.

Jing, qi, and shen are built on one another. Proficient jing leads to balanced qi. Balanced qi creates better shen. Improving the circulation of qi enhances and strengthens jing, as well as lifting shen. Good shen can control and connect to qi and be a guide to create more balanced qi. The cycle goes on and on, affecting each other in both positive and negative ways.

By practicing taiji and qigong, you strengthen the storage of jing, smooth the flow of the qi, and build better shen. You also improve physical health, psychological well-being, and expand and enhance the spirit.

During my many years of teaching, I have seen our students succeed in decreasing their stress level and increasing their overall health. They have made gains in flexibility, stamina, balance, poise, skill in interpersonal interactions, and mental focus.

The Benefits of Taiji in Four Major Parts
Physical

You will be enhancing your stamina and strength, building a balanced immune system and harmonized organ system, and preventing disease. From teaching taiji for more than thirty years, I have seen many students improve in their physical condition; they are sick less frequently even in flu season, they are physically stronger, and their chronic issues have improved. Many times, students have told me, "Everyone in my family gets sick except me," or they say, "I haven't been sick for several years." It is especially satisfying when I hear these things from senior citizens. It is easy to see that their overall health has improved, and some have even reduced their medications. There are more and more studies coming out on the benefits of taiji.

In the United States, scientists found that taiji clearly has benefits for the elderly in balance and preventing falls. This is just a side benefit of taiji. No doubt there will be more in-depth studies in the future on many of the important health benefits of taiji, such as preventing heart disease, reducing blood pressure, relieving depression and anxiety, and others.

Mental

Taiji definitely has the power to make you calm and less stressed. In my book *Tai Chi for Depression* (YMAA, 2017), I explain clearly how this works. In my experience, people who practice taiji over a lifetime tend to have fewer mental issues. Or if something dramatic happens, they know how to manage the stress.

Among the many antiaging benefits of taiji practice is mental clarity, which can bring improved reasoning and better efficiency in completing tasks. Your creativity is awakened, and you can make your life more multicolored and livelier. Your renewed alertness can help you keep relationships and friendships strong. As we have all experienced, it can be frustrating to have someone misunderstand what you are saying or to have to constantly remind someone about something—or frustrating to others when the person with the poor memory is you. Poor memory affects not only you but also the people who live with you, deal with you, and work with you on a daily basis. It might not bother you too much if you forget to do something someone asked you to do, but it may have been very important to the other person. Such situations and similar ones can strain relationships. This is my reason for teaching taiji and practicing it myself: to keep my own brain healthy. And it works. My memory is *better* than it was when I was younger.

Emotional

Practicing taiji balances the emotions, and the results are often immediate. People who seriously practice taiji tend to display an evenness of mood. They are able to better control their emotions during conflict and stressful situations. They let things go more easily. This is because of smooth energy flow in their organ system as well as the benefits to the brain. We will see more details on this in chapter 2 under the section named "How Taiji and Qigong Prevent Brain Aging and Memory Loss."

Spiritual

The spirit is that which is beyond the ordinary; it is an intangible, higher consciousness that never dies. It connects us with ourselves, both physically and emotionally. Spirit defines who we are, how we think, *what* we think, and how we interrelate with the universe. It also describes both how we view God and our relationship with God. Spirit is a special energy that cannot be seen, heard, touched, or otherwise experienced *materially*. It can, however, be felt or experienced *internally* by ourselves, by people around us, and even by animals. I have a dog, a lovely dog. When my spirit energy is poor, she can sense it. She comes to sit near me and tries to be very quiet. When my spirit energy is high, she wants to play. (Fortunately, my spirit energy is pretty good most of the time.) Our spirits are on a constant path toward enlightenment, constantly weighing, experiencing, and reacting to life's yin (receptive, dark, feminine) and yang (active, bright, masculine) sides.[2]

The meditative aspect of taiji allows us to tap into and activate our spirits. Our minds translate what our bodies feel as we move and interpret our spirits at the same time. Our minds integrate what we sense about the world in order to allow us to move our body accordingly. Taiji can also be said to be a way of expressing the spirit through the mind and body.

When we practice as a group, our spirits coalesce. Our spirits each accumulate the group energy, which we then express in unity or *as one*. But whether we practice taiji alone or with others, we are connecting body, mind, and spirit with the whole universe.

Taiji is known as a meditative art form. And like meditation, practicing taiji helps to balance the spirit as well as our own yin and yang aspects. We can then avoid being absorbed or overtaken by *negative* spirit or negative energy. It is as though taiji helps us to create a shield against negative energy. We tend to gravitate more toward people with positive spirit, and we more easily embrace positive spirit.

2. Please refer to my book *Simple Chinese Medicine* (YMAA, 2009) for information about yin and yang.

Mind, body, and spirit connect with one another in an important way. When you let your mind, body, and spirit work together, you are at peace with yourself. You become aware of your energy and feel the effects of taiji in your body. Additionally, you enjoy the sense of satisfaction that comes from performing the movements.

Daoist Practice

Taiji, qigong, and Chinese medicine all come from Daoist (also spelled Taoist) principles. In Daoist philosophy, everything on the earth has two opposite sides: yin and yang. To keep the balance of the cosmos, yin and yang must be balanced. In times of tragedy, chaos, and instability, as well as in cases of health problems, we will often see an imbalance of yin and yang. When practicing taiji, you are actually *walking the Daoist path*. Daoism helps you to be more relaxed, let go easier, and keep an inner peace. There are many versions of the *Dao De Jing* (often spelled *Tao Te Ching*) in bookstores. I recommend that you find a copy and read a chapter a day for bedtime learning.

Not Just for Senior Citizens: Taiji Is for Everyone

A common misconception I hear is that "taiji is for old people." Well, sure, many seniors are limited in what exercises they can do, and because taiji is slow, gentle, and has a very low risk of injury, it is ideally suited for seniors. But in truth, taiji is good for everyone, including children.

Learning taiji is actually a little easier for younger people, who can perform the more difficult movements, such as the stretching in the long lunges and the bending of the knees in the low stances. Older people will want to find an instructor with a great deal of experience teaching seniors and who knows how to modify the positions for their abilities. Seniors do not need to bend their knees as much, for example. They can just unlock their knees instead.

The main thing is that everyone who continues to practice taiji throughout their lives will see tangible results. You will notice that life seems easier, and your outlook is much more positive. Achievement will come more easily from having a well-balanced mind and body.

Many young people like to practice taiji so they can enhance their fighting abilities and power. There is great value in taiji as a martial art. Older people prefer to use taiji for fitness and longevity, to prevent an existing illness from getting worse, and to prevent illness from occurring. Still, you might see some older taiji practitioners who are practicing the martial aspects of this art as well.

Is Taiji a Real Workout?

Some people (both Chinese and American) complain that taiji seems too slow, that it doesn't look like it involves much physical exercise or have the feeling of a workout. This may be because the instructor did not give complete instructions or offer enough warm-up exercises. Maybe the students are not practicing long enough or following instructions well. Practicing taiji is very physical. You may be surprised at what a workout it is and how much physical power you can generate. Taiji's workout is invisible, subtle. It is slow for a reason—to develop concentration—but it has a power that is very strong and rooted. Patience and persistence are the keys to success in taiji.

In our modern, fast-paced society, we need a slow and balanced exercise to help regulate our lives. If we are busy all the time with no breaks or rest, our bodies will be overdriven, and just like an overused, unmaintained car, it will break down sooner than it should. When body chemicals like adrenaline and noradrenaline are at a high level for a long time, the heart gets overstimulated. In such a state, we are prone to heart disease, high blood pressure, and rapid aging. If we work our minds too hard, think too hard, or think every minute, our creativity and productivity slow down, and brain aging is likely. Nonstop or high-stress lifestyles invite many other problems, including high cholesterol, low energy problems, impaired immune function, cancer, and many others. A dog runs fast, and its life span is less than eighteen years. The turtle moves slowly, and its life span is around one hundred to one hundred fifty years, depending on its species. Perhaps there's a lesson to be drawn from this. The human life span can vary. How long do you want yours to be? The most important thing is not just to live longer but to live better. If I have a poor quality life, I don't need to live longer. But if I have a quality life, I want to enjoy it for as long as I can. By eating well, focusing on preventive work, and practicing taiji and qigong, you can prolong your life and constantly improve it.

Because taiji promotes internal strength by building strong qi, it can be a powerful training tool for martial artists. Many martial art schools offer taiji classes for both martial arts practitioners and nonpractitioners. You don't have to be a martial artist to benefit from taiji. People of all ages and abilities practice this exercise for all-around well-being exercise, including people with disabilities and other serious ailments.

How Taiji and Qigong Assist Human Healing

In the Chinese healing system, your mind and your body cannot be separated. Your body can affect your mind, and your mind can affect your body. Your energy pathways running through your body also run through your brain and affect all parts of the brain including the neurochemicals.

Both taiji and qigong work on internal energy. Internal energy brings harmony to the organ system. A harmonious organ system helps to balance biochemistry, hormones, and metabolism in the body. This is how your healing ability is enhanced. When you have surgery, your wound may be healed in days or weeks, even months. It all depends on your level of healing ability. When you catch a cold, you may recover in days, weeks, or months; this also depends on your healing ability. If your healing ability is strong, you can heal any illness. (I know some people don't believe this, especially medical people—I used to be one of them.) If your healing ability is poor or weak, your chance of healing is poor. It might take longer to heal, or you could even lose your life. Using taiji and qigong to improve your healing ability provides a powerful reason to start your taiji journey. Here is how taiji and qigong are associated with healing.

Cardiovascular Support

The slow and meditative movements of taiji and qigong help to smooth the flow of the energy. Taiji and qigong elevate the function of the vagus nerve system (involved in organ function), which has a big effect on reducing stress and preventing heart disease and hypertension. As we discussed previously, qi is the motor of the body. Just like a car, a bigger car with a bigger motor will go faster and have more power; a smaller car will go slower and have less power. If qi in the body is strong and balanced, your body and circulation system will be strong, and you will be less likely to develop circulatory and vascular diseases. For many years in China, the rates of heart disease and hypertension have been low. One of the reasons for this is that people pay attention to and work on improving their bodies' qi circulation. They also maintain a healthy diet, have a balanced and active social life, and often walk instead of drive. Recently, the situation has changed: there is now more heart disease, hypertension, diabetes, obesity, and other problems. There are also more cars now too, not surprisingly.

Respiratory Support

One of the most important benefits, which is also easy for Westerners to understand, is the increased oxygen level in the blood and organ system. Both taiji and qigong require deep breathing. With each slow and deep breath, you bring more oxygen to your body, to your lungs, and to your bloodstream. Your blood travels to all parts of the body. The more oxygen you bring into the body, the better your body's health.

Taiji and qigong not only increase the oxygen flow in the body but also increase its usage by organs and tissues. That is why taiji and qigong are considered natural antioxidants. This antioxidant property helps delay the aging process. By practicing deep breathing, your lung energy improves. To put it in Western terms, when lung capacity increases, we get more oxygen. On one trip to China, I had my friends examine my chest X-ray film. One friend practices internal medicine, and the other is a radiologist. Both of them told me it was amazing that even though I had chronic inflammation in my lungs, the amount of air I could breathe was remarkably good. I was disappointed about my inflammation—I was born with poor lung and kidney energy—but I was happy about my lung *function*. This helps bring a good amount of oxygen to my body. I am proof that people who have chronic lung issues can be helped with qigong and taiji.

These exercises also help to prevent respiratory infection, cold, flu, or any kind of lung disease. In our lungs, there are special antibodies called IgA (immunoglobulin A). IgA protects us from respiratory infection. Theoretically, qigong practice increases IgA in both quantity and quality. In Chinese medical theory, qigong practice improves your defensive energy, which is also called protective energy. People who practice qigong are less likely to get respiratory diseases and colds. I often feel blessed that I haven't been sick for many years.

Gastrointestinal Support

Taiji and qigong improve the autonomic nervous system, including both the sympathetic nervous system and the parasympathetic nervous system. In a later chapter, we will find out how important these nervous systems are to our health. The parasympathetic nerves are responsible for internal organs, especially the digestive system. With improved blood circulation, more oxygen gets to the organs. And with improved parasympathetic nerve function, the mobility of the digestive tract, your digestive enzymes, and other digestive chemicals are more likely to stay at healthy levels. When intestine mobility is normal, you have natural cleansing and detoxification.

You know you don't feel well if you cannot go to the bathroom for several days. Maintaining good digestive energy leads to better digestion and absorption. With these advantages, the food you eat will be properly used and transformed to energy. Otherwise, the food you eat will not be transformed to energy, and you will feel tired even though you may have eaten well. The movements in taiji and qigong involve the whole body, and sometimes you are in effect giving your internal organs a gentle massage during practice. This gentle stimulation helps to restore the balance of the digestive organs and prevent digestive disorder.

I have been surprised to find out that there are so many cases of digestive illness in the United States. I have many patients with digestive illnesses, very few of whom are willing to do taiji and qigong. But my patients who have taken my advice and practiced taiji and qigong did improve.

Many people take various supplements trying to help themselves. Supplements can help you if your digestive system can absorb and use them. But if you have imbalance in the digestive system, using supplements is rather wasteful because your supplements are not absorbed or used well either. True masters of taiji and qigong rarely have digestive problems. Diligent practice of taiji can help you to reach your goal of optimal health.

Musculoskeletal Support

Taiji and qigong involve the whole body with flexion, contraction, stretching, and multidimensional movements. Your muscles and joints are in constant motion and receive plenty of oxygen from the workout, making for a well-rounded form of exercise.

This not only keeps you fit but also keeps your muscles and joints healthy. You will have less muscle tension and stiffness. This helps delay aging and degeneration of the muscles and joints and maintains good muscle resiliency and flexibility. Healthy muscles and tendons can also prevent arthritis, fibromyalgia, and tendonitis. Not only will you have fewer aches and pains and less stiffness, but you will also have less chance of a fracture when you fall because strong and flexible muscles support your bones. Consequently, your body feels younger.

In 1991 I went to China. As usual, I went to a public park in the early morning and saw an eighty-two-year-old woman doing qigong. She kicked her leg even higher than I could. I then found out she came to this park to exercise every day, rain or shine.

I know it is easier to practice in China because there are so many people practicing in public parks. This, in itself, creates an energy field, and you spontaneously do it without hesitation. It is harder in America, not only because it is such a new thing here, but also because people feel self-conscious exercising in a public place. I think that is why we don't see many people doing these exercises outdoors.

Increase Stamina, Daily Energy Level, and Immune Function

Taiji strengthens the immune system. People who practice taiji not only improve their balance and coordination, but they also improve their immunity. A study from the Neuropsychiatric Institute at the University of California, Los Angeles, showed very interesting results in a group of older men and women who took taiji for forty-five minutes, three days a week.[3] The subjects showed an increase of up to 50 percent of memory T-cells. These are the immune system cells that identify and fight the varicella herpes virus, which causes shingles. People who have had chicken pox are vulnerable to shingles because the virus can remain dormant in nerve cells indefinitely. As we get older, our immune system gets weaker, so the virus can wake up. Shingles causes blisters on the skin and is very painful.

3. Michael R. Irwin, Jennifer L. Pike, Jason C. Cole, and Michael N. Oxman, "Effects of a Behavioral Intervention, Tai Chi Chih, on Varicella-Zoster Virus Specific Immunity and Health Functioning in Older Adults," *Psychosomatic Medicine* 65 (2003): 824–830. Results of the study were published in the September 2003 issue of *Psychosomatic Medicine*.

With improved energy flow, your body reaches an optimum state. Your endurance and stamina will be strong. You will be able to work longer hours and still have good productivity. Because of the balanced chemicals in the body, the immune system tends to be balanced too. People who practice taiji and qigong have much less chance of getting sick. In my teaching, I have seen many of my students improve their energy levels and immune systems. They rarely catch colds. Even when they have caught colds, they recovered more quickly than others.

Effects on the Nervous System

As mentioned above, the movements from taiji and qigong affect the nervous system, including the central nervous system, peripheral nervous system, and autonomic nervous system. The whole-body exercise incorporates breathing and mental focus, which allow qi and blood to flow better to all parts of the body, including the brain. By balancing the biochemicals and neurochemicals in the body and brain, you can be more focused, learn more quickly, think more logically, maintain mental sharpness and alertness, and improve your ability to perform daily tasks with greater ease.

Taiji and qigong not only regulate the somatic nervous system, as evidenced by the improved mobility of the muscles and joints, but also improve the autonomic nervous system, including sympathetic and parasympathetic nerve system response. The autonomic nervous system is divided into two opposite functions and is composed of the sympathetic and parasympathetic nervous systems. These neural networks control the internal organ systems, glands, blood vessels, and sensory systems. For many years, my focus has been on nervous system and autonomic healing. The healing work I do and the special exercises I create are designed to improve and balance the entire nervous system.

Each deep inhalation stimulates sympathetic activity, whereas each exhalation stimulates parasympathetic activity. The more regulated breathing you practice, the better-balanced autonomic nerve system you will have. That is why qigong masters have much fewer physical complaints in their lives. They tend to have a very good digestive function as well as a strong immune system. These are results of taiji and qigong's self-regulating effect on the human body.

There will be more details about the autonomic nervous system in a coming chapter, but suffice it to say here that these benefits remain even as you age, which has given me the encouragement to write this book. I have seen many of my friends with declining memories, even some who were very smart at a younger age. On the other hand, I have noticed that my taiji and qigong students have less depression and anxiety, stress, and confusion in making decisions. They greatly benefit people who have attention deficit disorder too. I believe if we start to teach children taiji or qigong at early ages, it could help them to focus, and they would do better in their academic studies and other activities. They would have healthier mental processes too.

Correction of Chemical Imbalances

Deep, slow, and regulated breathing helps to harmonize the body's chemistry, including adrenaline, noradrenaline, serotonin, and many other neurochemicals. Many illnesses are caused by chemical or hormonal imbalances. If you use external chemicals to balance the internal chemicals, such as taking a pill to supplement low levels of a chemical in the blood, you may actually cause more imbalances by interfering with the body's natural biofeedback response. Our bodies are autoregulating systems, which allow us to be in balance most of the time. If a certain chemical is low, the autoregulating system will stimulate the corresponding organ to release more of this particular chemical to balance the level. External chemicals (like pills) suppress this self-regulating response and provide false information to the body, so it stops releasing the very chemical it needs. That is why a person who takes a thyroid hormone pill, for example, will usually have to take it for life. If a person uses a pill to supplement the thyroid hormone, the destruction of the self-regulating system of the thyroid gland, pituitary gland, and hypothalamus will result; then his or her thyroid will no longer function. Conversely, if those with thyroid problems practice taiji or qigong consistently or get acupuncture or Chinese herb treatments instead, they have a chance of restoring the self-regulating system. Eventually, the level of the hormones will become normal.

With taiji and qigong practice, there is definitely a feeling of chemical balance. There is stillness in motion, and there is motion in stillness. If it involved just stillness without any motion, it might be difficult for some people to follow. If it were just motion without stillness, such as a heavy workout offers, we would lose the sense of peace and harmony. Try to practice taiji and qigong when you are stressed and see how you feel afterward.

Other Benefits

- Improved metabolism: You rarely see an overweight qigong master or longtime practitioner.

- Improved balance and coordination: Research has shown balance and coordination help to prevent falls and injuries.

- Improvement in quality of life and happiness: This is from becoming well balanced and open minded. The masters of taiji and qigong don't get stressed because they know how to avoid negative energy.

- Improved learning ability in all fields: We will have more details on this in later chapters.

- Harmony in the working of the organs: This is obviously very important in health and healing. Please reference my book *Simple Chinese Medicine* for information regarding organ teamwork.

- Cancer healing: Taiji and qigong help prevent cancer and cancer relapse. They can also help to heal cancer. I know very few people believe this statement. A majority of people might say, "Yeah right, Doc, this is a joke. Cancer needs chemotherapy, radiation therapy, hormone therapy, steroid therapy, surgery, and drugs." Sound familiar? But think for a moment: how many cancer patients die even though they receive these conventional therapies? Common sense shows a balanced mind leads to a balanced body, and a balanced body helps you to heal. Anything can change: your health, your illness, your life too. I could be crippled by my chronic lung inflammation by now, but I am not.

Taiji and qigong strengthen the immune system, and a strong immune system helps to fight cancer. People who have a strong immune system tend to die from old age even if they have cancer cells in their bodies. Only if you have a weak immune system can the cancer cells grow faster and be more invasive. A weakened immune system caused by some conventional treatments can cause severe infection, which is a main cause of death for cancer patients. Taiji and qigong can put patients into a positive state of mind and promote positive thoughts, giving crucial hope for healing. Scientists know the mind has immense power with regard to human disease and healing. I have seen this firsthand.

In China, people who have cancer always seek treatment from both medicines: conventional and holistic. Most of them do qigong regularly in addition to using herbal medicine. I have several cancer patients who visit me regularly, and they are doing very well. I highly recommend that if you have cancer, start to use qigong or taiji as a lifetime companion. You will not regret it.

Please keep in mind taiji and qigong are not magic, even though they can provide amazing benefits. All the benefits come from diligent practice, faith, a positive attitude, and patience.

Taiji, the True Art of Healing and Well-Being

As I mentioned earlier, when I was starting out as a doctor, my focus was mainly on treating disease. Now, my focus is on teaching people how to prevent disease. This may not seem that impressive (no one appreciates good health when everything seems fine). But it has incredible value, as anyone can appreciate when they see others suffering from serious illness. I have always believed that prevention should be the job of a good doctor. I believe this is what gives a doctor value as a health-care provider. I have come by this belief about good health from my lifetime of practice and from teaching and training people in taiji and qigong.

Chapter 3

Taiji and Brain Fitness

Have you seen my watch?
Have you seen my wallet?
What time is my appointment again?
Where did I put my papers?
I cannot find my keys.
I cannot find my checkbook.
I forgot to go to my class.
I forgot all about my appointment today.
What were you saying?
I cannot find my red shirt.
Where is my cell phone?

Sound familiar? If thoughts like these don't characterize you, they surely characterize people you know—and maybe you someday. Our brains start aging at around age twenty-four. It is widely believed that we lose many neurons every year as we age (some say one hundred thousand—that's a scary thought). When we have difficulty with perception and memory, we get frustrated, anxious, and even depressed. When we forget something important, it costs us money, time, and energy. In some cases, it can be very disturbing.

Many years ago, a friend of mine was going on a trip. He needed to fly to Germany for work. When he went to check in at the airport, he realized that he had forgotten to bring his airplane ticket and his photo ID. He had to drive forty miles back home to pick them up because at the time there was no electronic ticketing. Of course, he missed the plane and had to take a later one. What if there had been only one flight that day, or if he'd had an engagement he couldn't miss? Another friend of mine forgot to turn off the stove one day. She accidentally started an oil fire and burned a kitchen cabinet. This obviously could have been much worse. My family and friends have many stories about umbrellas left behind in stores; watches, wallets, or jewelry left on hotel bedside tables; credit cards left in restaurants; or being unable to find tickets for a show.

I am not saying I am perfect, but I am aware of when things need to be worked on and try to take action accordingly. I have seen the difference a proactive approach to brain antiaging has made in my own life. Many people feel that their memory is getting worse, but I am happy to say mine is just fine. It is as strong as it was twenty years ago even though I am sure I have lost many brain cells due to aging like any older person.

The sad part is that forgetfulness seems to be a problem for younger and younger people, even teenagers. Maybe this is from our busy lifestyle or from having too much on our plates. Maybe we are not pointing our brains in the right direction. Or we could be too conservative and unwilling to change. Maybe we just cannot focus. Kids or younger people could be using too many electronics instead of using their brains. Or maybe some people are just born with poor memories.

Everything has two sides. We tend to be more forgetful when we get older, but getting older also has benefits. We are wiser, more mature, more experienced, and have a better understanding of life. We are more willing to improve and overcome our weaknesses, including poor memory. I have always believed that anything is possible. We should keep in mind that anything can change, and anything can improve.

I used to be very forgetful in my younger days due to inherited weak kidney qi. I remember how much I struggled due to my poor health when I was in medical school. I struggled to memorize and comprehend the material. In my early years, sometimes I couldn't remember if I'd locked my office door, so I'd have to drive back to the office. Several times, I got back to the office and found that the door was unlocked. This gave me the desire to improve my brain and my memory. I will share with you how I did that with taiji and qigong. But first, let's begin with a basic understanding of our brains.

Understanding Our Brains and Brain Aging

The brain is a special organ with a very complicated wiring system similar to a computer network. This three-pound lump of wrinkled tissue with no observable moving parts directs all parts of the body, including all movement, sensation, thought processing, creativity, emotion, talking, eating, walking, self-regulating, breathing, and much more.

Our brains are complex and mysterious and present a multitude of challenges to understanding how it works. It is so advanced and interesting that it makes us want to explore more. The chemistry in the brain is also very complex. It enables hundreds of different personalities and various emotions to be expressed.

Scientists are finding out new things about it every day. The medical and pharmaceutical industries also study the brain to help them create new drugs to change our brain chemistry and treat mental illness and brain degeneration. Educators study the brain in hopes of finding ways to improve learning skills in children and younger adults. I study the brain mainly to improve my own memory and enjoyment of life. Although we may never completely unravel the mystery of the brain, we have learned much about it.

Let's look briefly at the construction of the organ itself.

The Three Major Parts of the Brain

The brain consists of three main parts: the forebrain, the midbrain, and the hindbrain. The forebrain is made up of the cerebrum, thalamus, and hypothalamus (the hypothalamus is part of the limbic system, which is involved in memory, learning, emotion, and motivation). The midbrain is the smallest part that helps relay auditory and visual information. The hindbrain includes most of the brainstem and the cerebellum, among other parts. The brainstem is responsible for very basic functions like breathing and the beating of the heart, while the cerebellum is associated with movement, special perception, and balance.

Brain Hemispheres

The brain is divided into two halves: the left brain hemisphere and the right brain hemisphere. The left brain controls the right side of the body, and the right brain controls the left side of the body. Although they mirror each other in appearance, they govern different intellectual and physical functions.

For a long time, the left brain hemisphere was thought of as the most important side, whereas the right brain hemisphere was considered somewhat less important. But the reality is that both sides of our brains are equally important. Most people have dominance on one side or the other. They are either left-brain dominant or right-brain dominant. Few people have both sides of the brain with equal strength. Some people know they have a dominant side and pay special attention to strengthening both sides of their brains. Those who pay attention to strengthening both sides are considered really smart and intelligent. It seems these people, who work on enhancing both sides are less easily confused, have less sickness, and fewer problems in their lives. Also, these people have a better chance of succeeding in their undertakings, the goals they want to achieve, and maintaining relationships.

Functionality and Characteristics Attributed to the Left and Right Hemispheres

Research carried out by Dr. Robert Ornstein (University of California) found that the left brain handles these mental activities:

- Mathematics

- Language

- Logic

- Analysis

- Writing

- Other similar activities

The right brain handles different activities:

- Imagination

- Color

- Music

- Rhythm

- Daydreaming

- Other similar activities[4]

From the above lists, it appears the logical, objective left brain fits more with Western philosophy or culture, whereas the intuitive, subjective right brain fits more

4. Tony Buzan, *Make the Most of Your Mind* (New York: Simon & Schuster, 1984), 23.

with Eastern philosophy or culture. There are certainly many great scientists and inventors in the United States and more than enough artists and craftspeople in China. But according to Daoist philosophy and yin and yang theory, there is no absolute category for either one. Yin and yang can change, transform, and communicate. Yin and yang supplement and assist each other. They complement, support, and rely on each other. The brain is the same way. Its function can change and transform. The two sides of the brain can assist, complement, support, and rely on each other. The weaker side of your brain can be strengthened by proper training. This is referred to as neuroplasticity. Tony Buzan, author of *Make the Most of Your Mind*, reports that Dr. Robert Ornstein "also found that people who had been trained to use one side of their brain more or less exclusively were relatively unable to use the other side, both in general and in specific situations where activities were related to the other side of the brain. He also found that when the 'weaker' of the two hemispheres was stimulated and encouraged to work in cooperation with the stronger side, the result was a great increase in overall ability and effectiveness."[5]

Most of us were taught to believe that strong left-brainers do well with reading, writing, and arithmetic, while right-brainers excel in art, music, and spatial reasoning. This kind of thinking uses outdated findings and theories to put people into a box, insisting that a strongly right-brain person has less of a chance at succeeding in science or business, whereas the common sense and intuition of a left-brain person are thought to be automatically weaker. But this is really too simplistic. Our brains are not completely separated. The right brain is just as important as the left brain for proper cognitive functioning.

Because our two brains are connected through the corpus callosum, a large bundle of nerve fibers connecting the two cerebral hemispheres, the two brains can cooperate to do similar work, and the weak brain can become stronger through training. If we train ourselves to work with both sides of the brain and give them enough stimulation, we can achieve a great deal no matter which side of the brain may be stronger.

This explains why the brain will benefit from taiji practice and learning. The 360-degree movements in space force your right and left hemispheres to communicate

5. Ibid.

back and forth, trading off dominance in a continuous, integrated exercising of the brain and body. We will discuss this in detail later.

Eastern and Western Brains

What I call the "Eastern brain" refers to the typical Asian way of processing or doing things, or generally approaching life from the standpoint of Eastern philosophy. Of course, the Eastern brain may not necessarily characterize a westernized Asian person's way of approaching things any more than every citizen of the West always has a "Western brain." Many Asians have assimilated Western cultural ideas very successfully, and many Westerners have adopted Asian cultural ideas with aplomb as well. It is certainly clear from my recent visits to China that the Chinese culture is becoming westernized in some areas, just as we see evidence of Asian cultural influences here in the United States. Perhaps we are moving toward a global, balanced brain. We'll see.

Here are some examples of the behavioral differences between the so-called Western and Eastern brains. These examples are meant to illustrate rather than be definitive. And again, they are not meant to imply that one is better than the other or that all people of a particular race or culture exhibit these same qualities. There are no absolutes.

Cooking

The traditional Western style of cooking is to follow a recipe that lists the exact ingredients, quantities, cooking method, temperature, special equipment needed, and so on. Even when trying to learn from friends or family, most people ask, "Would you please give me the recipe?" The Asian style of cooking, in contrast, uses general varieties and amounts of ingredients such as salt, pepper, soy sauce, vinegar, ginger, garlic, and hot pepper to create many different dishes. When trying to learn a new dish from friends or family, they get the main ingredients and general instructions from conversation and then follow their own taste for the specifics.

Traveling or Vacationing

Many Western travelers like to plan far in advance, scheduling flights, booking hotels, buying tickets for attractions, and making restaurant reservations well ahead of embarking on their trips. Many Asian travelers, on the other hand, go places when they feel like it, mapping the route as they go, and staying at whatever hotel they find along the way. However, as the wealthy middle class continues to grow in China and as time becomes scarcer with work schedules, their approach to making holiday plans will likely become more westernized.

Disease and Healing

In the West, most disease diagnosis involves conducting tests on the patient to isolate the cause, interpreting the results, and making treatment recommendations aimed at specific symptoms. The effectiveness of a treatment is measured by lab tests or with other technological means. The Eastern approach views disease as an imbalance and stagnation of energy flow. Healing work focuses on correcting the root of the problem and allowing the person to heal him- or herself. Evaluations of treatment are based on what patients report about their overall feeling, as well as the healer's own assessment. This makes the quality of the practitioner very important.

Values

Traditional Western values, in general, tend to lean very much toward materialism. This is related to the capitalist economic system. Traditional Eastern values often lean more toward the values of family life, harmony, the search for balance in one's life, and personal well-being. Today, many people from the East and West are blending both traditions in a search for the best of both.

Regulations

Westerners follow rules very well. Yes means yes and no means no. In the East, many people follow the rules well only to a certain degree. Sometimes, to some people, yes can change to no, and no can change to yes depending on the situation. I call this elasticity.

Working

In the West, in many cases the company is the main structure for conducting business, often with a management team led by a CEO, a detailed organizational structure, modern information technology systems, and controls for achieving the firm's objectives.

The ownership of the company is often through its shareholders if the company is public. In the East, many companies are still owned and run by a patriarch and his family. This again is changing as more companies go public in Asia. However, in the West, it is clear that separating ownership from management does not always lead to the best decisions being made for the company or its shareholders. There is something to be said for Western management behaving more like owners of a company rather than as temporary tenants. Eastern workers, however, seem more loyal to the company and more willing to work hard. This may have something to do with the competition and huge population.

Lifestyle and Financial Planning

Most people in the West plan ahead for retirement whereas in traditional Eastern culture the tendency is to save money for the children until they are well established. As long as they're not yet standing on their own two feet, the family may continue to support them. I have seen many Asians who saved money their whole lives while maintaining poor lifestyles but nonetheless left money to their children when they died. Fortunately, in most Asian families, the children also take care of their parents when the parents are older, disabled, or have some medical issue that requires assistance.

Dealing with People

Westerners often express things directly, making their viewpoint clear, whereas in the East, people express things less straightforwardly. Sometimes you might even have to guess what the speaker really means. This can sometimes cause confusion and misunderstanding.

Activities

Popular Western culture encourages thrill-seeking behavior as people search for excitement and that rush of adrenaline, whereas in Eastern cultures, contemplation, peace, tranquility, quiet, stillness, and calm continue to be valued.

Because the world is changing, tradition and culture everywhere are also changing. People are getting smarter and trying to learn whatever is good for their lives. I've lived in the United States for more than twenty years, and I've seen many people living their lives in a traditional way. Still others try to make their lives better with a balance of tradition and change.

A long-term patient of mine named John used to be so stubborn and stiff in his ways. He is a brilliant man and very analytical about everything. Working with him was a challenge for me. I was trying to help him with his many physical ailments and also trying to educate him about Daoist philosophy, which could offer him new skills for stress management and relaxation. I also gave him some extra homework to help him to balance both sides of his brain. Because of his stubbornness and highly stressed personality, he was suffering from serious heart disease and hypertension. In Chinese medicine, the mind is closely related to heart energy. This explains why so many people with long-term stress are prone to heart disease and heart attacks. After working with him for a year using multiple approaches, his heart condition improved, his attitude improved, and he became much more relaxed and easygoing. He was finally able to see things from multiple angles. Perhaps the biggest highlight was that his relationship with his family improved. The Western mind can benefit from Eastern ways and insights, just as the Eastern mind can benefit from Western influences.

Brain Aging and Brain Antiaging

Many holistic health practitioners use their knowledge and experience with the brain, mind, and awareness to guide patients to heal themselves in their healing work. In my practice with natural healing and natural medicine, I have seen many miracles; it is as if anything is possible if you put enough effort, intent, and energy into the work. The many cases of healing from cancer are especially important examples of the power of this mind-body approach.

The brain is composed of some one hundred billion cells called neurons. The neuron, unlike other cells, has many arms or branches like an octopus. These millions of branches are like tentacles radiating in all directions. The tentacles are called dendrites. Each of these dendrites has thousands of tiny protuberances, much like the suction pads on the tentacles of the octopus but protruding from all sides. These form communication pathways between nerve cells that form the basis of learning and memory.

In the past, intelligence was thought to be related to the number of brain cells and poor memory to the loss of brain cells. We also believed brain cells could not be replaced. But scientists have now determined that the adult brain not only can grow new cells but can also sprout new dendrites. Scientists know now that it is not the number of the brain cells that determines a person's intelligence, but rather intelligence is associated with the protuberances on the brain cells' tentacles. Crossing the protuberances of each brain cell, electrochemical impulses form patterns with individual cells and groups. To put it another way, it is like a human social network: if you know one person, you may learn something from that one person. And if you know many different people and communicate with them all, you may learn a lot more. These dendrites on the nerve cells receive and process information from other nerve cells, thus forming the basis of memory. When our minds are underused or inadequately challenged, we risk losing a great deal of our brainpower. If the dendrites don't communicate regularly, they can atrophy. This reduces the ability to put new information into memory and makes it difficult to retrieve old information. This also reduces other brain functioning such as cognitive ability, spatial orientation, and logical ability.

It is usually assumed that the brain declines with age. This decline is supposed to include memory, attention span, mathematical ability, creativity, alertness, learning ability, and language. It is said that once you reach a certain age, your ability to grow and learn new things bottoms out—"you can't teach an old dog new tricks." But that's wrong. New data indicate you *can* teach an old dog new tricks *if* the old dog is willing to learn. It is true that our bodies degenerate with age. But the brain is not the same; this mysterious organ does not get old side by side with the body. New findings from science show that if the brain is consistently stimulated, no matter at what age, it can remain young and healthy. It doesn't matter if you are forty or seventy. When stimulated through various activities, the brain will generate new connections far more rapidly on average than it will lose brain cells. Keep this in mind: it's the connections and the communication between the brain cells that keeps our brains young, keeps our memory working, makes our brains function well, and keeps us intelligent and creative. Many experts agree that the adult brain can actually *improve* with age, and this has been demonstrated through scientific study.

The human brain is a biological supercomputer. Even though we have learned a great deal of information about the brain to date, there is so much more for us to explore.

How Taiji and Qigong Prevent Brain Aging and Memory Loss

As we age, our bodies slow down, and we tend to become forgetful. The good news is that research has shown that it is possible to maintain and even restore our memory function and learning ability. I have been experimenting with ways of doing this my whole life in an effort to support my health, my learning ability, my overall improvement, and my memory. My goal is to avoid dementia and physical disability and be able to enjoy my life for as long as I can.

Practicing taiji and qigong is very effective in preventing physical decline and brain aging. Over the centuries, countless people have used these arts to improve their physical and mental health. Over time, what has no value is left behind, and what has value is retained. From thousands of years of experience, the Chinese know what methods are effective for achieving good health, and they use them. In the West, on the other hand, people seem to require scientific evidence for everything. For instance, I would guess that many people living a Daoist lifestyle in China would be hard put to explain the Dao. Some of them probably don't even know what the Dao is. Recently, more and more research has been done to support Daoist conceptions scientifically, so perhaps people are becoming better educated about it. But they made great practical use of the philosophy of the Dao even before.

The use of taiji and qigong to prevent brain aging is presented here from my own experience, including the changing behavior and attitudes seen in my students, as well as the observations of many masters. I have summarized this way of using taiji and qigong in the following fourteen points.

1. Lifelong Learning

Learning should never stop. I always tell my family—and say the same thing in my lectures and other speaking engagements—"the day you stop learning is the day you stop living." Learning is a big part of healing; healing is a big part of learning. Taiji involves learning. When you start to learn things you didn't know, you begin to shift your focus to new knowledge, new approaches, new movements, and a new lifestyle. Taiji learning is continuous and multileveled in skill, depth, and meaning. Through continuous learning and practice, you will get the meaningful part—the true nature of taiji. If you are just starting as a beginner, you will feel good immediately from the practice of relaxation. If you are an advanced student, you will feel good continuously from the sustained practice of energy fluidity. Either way, you get benefits. Even people who do it incorrectly still get benefits. As you practice for more than a year or two, your taiji form will become more graceful and beautiful, and you will feel like you are dancing on the clouds. This gives you an added feeling of accomplishment and satisfaction. Learning taiji is challenging, but the challenge will help you enhance brain plasticity, which will support you as you age.

Any kind of challenge is stimulation for our brains. Without challenge, we would never be able to invent things. Without challenge, our lives would not advance. If we rely on a calculator all the time, soon we can't calculate easy equations anymore. If we store every phone number in our cell phone contacts list or computer, we won't be able to dial those numbers ourselves. In one scientific study on aging and the brain, scientists confirmed that *any* intellectually challenging activity and *any* activity involving mildly complex movement stimulate the growth of dendrites, and this adds more connections in the brain's neural pathways.

When you work on learning taiji or qigong, you are shifting gears to a higher level of positive energy. The more positive energy you have, the more improvement you will see in all aspects of your life and being. The positive energy also goes to your brain, and therefore all of your body's parts function better.

Just as there are two halves of the brain, there are two types of thought: conscious and unconscious. Conscious thought involves your awareness of your surroundings, your agenda for the day, plans for work or travel, your pleasures, and your peeves. You can logically rearrange, discuss, and guide your behavior according to your needs. Unconscious thoughts, on the other hand, are more spontaneously occurring and out of your intentional control, such as holding a cup, saying goodnight to your spouse, and your heart beating fast when you are nervous. Taiji practice raises the quality of your conscious thought processes, empowering you to be more in tune with your daily experiences.

2. A Break in Your Routine

We grow up with certain fixed routines, and most of us don't want to change those routines. Such routines can include our diet, how we do our jobs, and the way we interact with people but also habitual ways of thinking. We don't like to do something if we are not familiar with it. While on a hiking trip with my sister and my husband in Acadia National Park, we got disoriented in the woods. My sister and I wanted to explore for a way out, but my husband insisted that we go back the same way to get out. Seeing his anxiety, I almost gave up and agreed to go back the same way. Suddenly, my sister found a new path. It guided us onto another main path, and we found our way back. She broke the routine and helped us find a new path out of the woods. We drive on the same road every day because the familiarity of the road is comforting. But if we never try a different road, we'll never find a better route. Sometimes new roads are shortcuts or help us avoid traffic jams.

Routines can be brain deadening. When something unusual happens that gets us out of our routine, we get anxious; we don't know what to do. We feel like our brains are not working. Just think, many of us go to work every day, come home, eat, sleep, go to work the next day—our brains are programmed in such a way that we don't even have to think anymore. Our brain cells don't get stimulated and certain neural pathways shut down. *Breaking the routine is a brain fitness workout.* This allows new activities for the brain to be activated and encourages brain cells to communicate, opening new neural pathways. Watching TV is another brain-killing activity; however, this doesn't mean we need to give up on TV. I like to watch the news, some nature programs, and other educational programs. But research has shown that when we watch TV, the brain is less active, even less active than during sleep. When you are watching TV, your brain is passive—or active in a passive way. Some TV programs can even traumatize the brain, which can make us unable to view things as a whole. If you know how to balance your life, you will be careful to watch TV wisely and add other brain fitness exercises into your life. Think for a moment: how many smart couch potatoes are there? (I don't mean to say that all people who watch TV are couch potatoes, though.)

Taiji exercise and learning are not familiar to most Americans. We did not grow up with slow-motion exercises. We like fast and vigorous. We like *pain*. We often hear, "No pain, no gain." This is not an entirely accurate statement. Not all that long ago, human beings may have had to struggle just to survive. But things are different now; we don't have to suffer too much to get what we need. Our needs now go beyond surviving and just making a living. Physical burdens have been replaced with mental ones. We need tools to help us to relieve these mental burdens. In other words, even exercise in this modern lifestyle should be balanced—fast *and* slow movements. The yin energy (receptive, slow) and the yang energy (active, fast) should be evident everywhere to keep our lives balanced. Many of our problems are caused by the imbalance of yin and yang.

Once you open your mind, you can purposely disrupt your routine and adjust your old habits. You can build brain cells by choosing to experience a totally new concept, a new philosophy, a new way of life, a new journey. Your brain cells will have to branch out to make new connections with other brain cells.

I keep saying that taiji is a journey. That's because you are always learning new things from taiji practice, acquiring new knowledge, experiencing new sensations, making new movements or understanding old movements more deeply, and perhaps forging new friendships. Taiji opens your mind and shows you a pathway to a new way of seeing things.

3. Better, Deeper Sleep

We know sleeping disorders can accelerate aging, especially brain aging. The first thing you notice about people with sleep problems is that they look tired. The next thing you notice is that their speech is slow. This indicates that the brain language center is sluggish and less active. The same is true for other parts of the brain. We have all had the experience that if we don't sleep well the previous night, our minds are not clear, our memory is not sharp, and we cannot concentrate. The sleep-deprived brain has less ability to store new information and retrieve old information. I struggled with a sleeping disorder in medical school. This couldn't have helped my memory problems. The day I graduated, I said to myself, *I never want to go back to school again*, even though I hadn't done poorly at all.

Many of my patients with sleeping problems tell me, "My brain is in a fog" or "I can't remember things." If a person has had a long-term sleeping disorder, you can see that she looks older than she actually is. A good night's sleep is also an important part of healing from many illnesses. Just think about a machine: if used nonstop, the machine soon breaks down.

With regular practice of taiji and qigong, your neurochemicals are brought into balance, and your body's electricity and sleep become regulated. Your brain is no longer exhausted, and you are more alert. Now brain healing can begin.

4. Increased Oxygen

I mention oxygen so many times in my lectures, classes, trainings, short talks, and conversations. This is because it is so important to life and health. The brain, although only about 2 percent of your body weight, consumes roughly 20 percent of the oxygen you breathe in! When the brain is nurtured with adequate oxygen, it helps to bring better function to the respiratory and vascular centers and vice versa. If you have problems with your heart and lungs that affect your oxygen level, it will also affect the oxygen level in your brain. Cognitive power declines when there is a decreased supply of oxygen to the brain.

When I see a person yawning a lot, I tease him and say, "You need more oxygen." When I see someone who sleeps too much, I say, "You need more oxygen." When I see someone who is driving and feeling sleepy, I say, "You need more oxygen." If someone's tired: "You need more oxygen." Oh boy, if your energy is flagging, you better not be near me! When it comes to oxygen, I am a nagging mother.

As we know, the brain must consume oxygen to be able to function. It is the lungs that help us get oxygen through the breath. If your brain lacks oxygen for six to nine minutes, your brain can be damaged. If you lack oxygen for twenty minutes, you will die. If your body lacks food for fifteen days, you may still live. The oxygen to our brain is very important. If your brain has enough oxygen, you are most likely alert; if your brain lacks oxygen, you feel tired, lethargic, and overwhelmed by the mental fog. You will also notice that when you are tired or feel sleepy, you feel a little clearer after a big yawn. Yawning is the deepest breath we can take; we do it to get oxygen to our tired brains.

Adequate oxygen intake is crucial for preventing brain aging. Practicing qigong and taiji involves deep breathing, which helps to bring more oxygen to your body and your brain; you will notice the change in the way you feel overall. You will feel less cloudy, fresher, more alert, and more energetic.

5. Unique Taiji Movement Sequences

Taiji movements are not like any other exercise. The special choreographed movements are circular and in constant motion. Many gestures cross the body from left to right, from upward to downward, and from right diagonal to left diagonal. It is multidimensional. The footwork is slow, on the diagonal, well controlled, and involves multiple changing stances. Through these changing stances and whole-body movements, multidimensional both spatially and the internally, you learn to be more aware of your body. You become aware of your tension, your balance, your energy, your emotional stability, and your visual surroundings. You pay attention to your energy center and are able to self-correct your posture. You know if you are off-center or if you lose your balance. You move with your intention, and you move your body while your mind experiences calm and peace.

Taiji movement stimulates the senses, the faculty of motor control, the sense of spatial orientation, the sense of balance and equilibrium, the forebrain and hindbrain, and the left and right brain. It also provides cross-brain stimulation. The whole brain is stimulated. Taiji movements are very good brain fitness exercises. We use aerobic exercise to increase our heart rate and promote better circulation. We also need brain fitness exercises to improve our brain function and learning abilities. Western science has confirmed that movement is crucial to brain health and definitely affects cognitive change. Eastern practitioners knew it all along.

Evidence shows that movement is also crucial to every other brain function, including memory, emotion, language, learning, and more. Try to do qigong for three to five minutes when you are tired after working, or writing a paper if you are a student, and your brain can't seem to think anymore. You will be able to return to work refreshed or put more words on paper. What is happening here? Our higher brain functions evolved from lower functions involving basic mobility, and these higher functions still depend on the lower ones. A sedentary lifestyle promotes brain aging—too much TV or any other couch potato, "brain dead" activity.

The well-known kinesiology and learning researcher Dr. Paul Dennison, along with his wife, movement educator Gail Dennison, have developed a movement program that has been proven to exercise the brain. They call it Brain Gym. Brain Gym is a movement-based technique to enhance learning ability for children who have learning difficulties in conventional settings. As we age, we do not learn as quickly or as well as younger people. The information takes longer to put into memory storage, and it takes longer to learn new things. Studies have shown that we shift from being visual and auditory learners to *kinesthetic* learners. That is, we don't absorb so much from reading or listening as we once did—we need to learn by doing. Above and beyond this learning style, Brain Gym has helped to establish even stronger links between certain kinds of movement techniques and enhancing brain function in general. The exercise movements from taiji and qigong can help adults achieve maximum learning and delay the brain-aging process.

I have a friend named Nancy. Nancy's husband has several electronic systems hooked into the television and therefore needs several different remotes. To watch TV, she has to press numerous buttons on each remote. Even though her husband has taught her several times, she still cannot find the right button to turn on the TV. Finally, she just bought another TV with only one remote. Many older people have trouble using multisystem entertainment centers. Here is an opposite story. One of my taiji students studied piano at the age of fifty-eight. She told me that her piano teacher was amazed at her ability to learn. My own experience was learning cello—I didn't start until I was forty-nine. I was skeptical myself! But now I realize I can learn, and I even improve. It makes me feel good to see that improvement.

With certain body movements to stimulate neural pathways, you enable nerve cells to communicate with each other and create more activity in the brain network. The participant feels more alert and can easily put memory into storage and later retrieve the information. That is why we say taiji enhances learning ability.

Taiji and qigong movements balance both sides of the brain by encouraging cross-connections with information between the left and right brain. With this special training, our dominant side can become more cooperative with the other, fostering a greater balance between the two sides. This hemispheric balance helps you to develop well-balanced cognitive, communication, and social skills. Once your brain is more balanced, you may even be more pleasant with your partner or companion, more easy-going, better able to multitask, more even-tempered, have an increased ability to learn new things, and be less rigid or stubborn. These are some of the changes I have observed firsthand in many of my students.

The cross-brain movements create a sort of cross-brain training. The stimulation causes more communication to occur through synapses of the brain cells. This enhanced connection and communication between the brain cells keeps our brains young and our memory strong.

Science has also confirmed that taiji improves the body's balance. The cerebellum controls balance, coordination, adjustment, and smoothing out of movement. Taiji improves the cerebellum's function, bringing about better coordination and balance.

Recent studies have shown that the cerebellum is not just related to movement but also to cognition. For those with injuries to the brain and cerebellum, there are studies that suggest a possibility for healing from taiji and qigong practice. Because taiji improves cerebellum function, it is likely practice of the art will improve both physical balance and cognitive skill. By rewiring the brain itself, not only can the brain learn new tricks, but it can also change its structure and function, even in old age. Taiji is truly a brain fitness regimen for adults.

6. Balance and the Autonomic Nerve System

In the human body, all functions are controlled through the nervous system, and all organs are controlled by the autonomic nerve system. Many illnesses are caused by disorders of these systems. My main focus in my healing work is regulating the nervous system, which made a big difference in my healing ability.

Understanding the Nervous System

Autonomic nerve impulses originate in the central nervous system and perform the most basic human functions automatically, without conscious control. Autonomic nerve fibers exiting from the central nervous system form the sympathetic, the parasympathetic, and the enteric nervous systems. The actions of the sympathetic and parasympathetic systems often oppose each other. For example, sympathetic nerves are responsible for increasing the heart rate, raising blood pressure, and causing us to breathe harder. The parasympathetic nerves do the opposite: decrease heart rate, reduce blood pressure, and slow down breath. The sympathetic system is involved in "fight and flight" responses while the parasympathetic division is involved in "rest and digest" actions that do not require an immediate response.

The sympathetic nervous system connects the internal organs to the brain. It responds to stress by increasing heart rate and blood flow to the muscles and decreasing blood flow to the skin. The parasympathetic nervous system increases digestive secretions and slows the heartbeat. Both systems give feedback to the central nervous system about the condition of internal organs to help maintain the body's equilibrium.

The autonomic nervous system controls the iris and the muscles involved in the functioning of the heart, lungs, stomach, and other organs. It is in charge of the automatic functions—those we have no control over. These include the beating of the heart, digestion, breathing, and sexual arousal. Emotions strongly influence the autonomic nervous system. For example, anger makes your heart beat faster, and anxiety can interfere with digestion.

Patients visit their doctors for unexplained symptoms, and they are disappointed when doctors cannot find anything wrong and cannot help them. These unexplained ailments are most likely caused by disorders of the autonomic nervous system. When I correct the imbalance of an autonomic disorder, the patient's symptoms diminish, and the patient feels better. When they call me a "miracle worker," I just tell them what I did: regulated autonomic function. The autonomic nervous system has a close relation to the meridian system in Chinese medicine. I love working with the nervous systems, especially the autonomic nervous system because people can feel the difference right away.

The movements in taiji and qigong, as well as total-body warm-up exercises, involve twisting and turning of the whole body, loosening the spine and all of the vertebrae joints. This makes these paired nerves work in harmony, balancing the autonomic nervous system and therefore maintaining homeostasis in the body and brain. Deep and slow breathing stimulate the respiratory and circulatory centers in the brain, helping to regulate autonomic function.

7. Building Qi, Harmonizing Energy

Qi is vital energy or life force. It is the energy that underlies everything in the universe. Qi in the human body refers to the various types of bioenergy associated with human health and vitality. Changing qi in our body can affect our health and well-being. Qi is present internally and externally and controls the function of all parts of the body. There are many different types of qi in the body. These are discussed in my book *Natural Healing with Qigong* (YMAA, 2004).

Taiji and qigong strengthen all of the organs—kidneys, heart, liver, spleen, and lungs. In traditional Chinese medicine, the kidney system is related to the brain. The heart system is related to shen (spirit) and also to the brain. The liver system is related to emotions and moods and is also associated with the brain. The spleen system is linked to digestion, absorption, metabolism, and blood—all bringing nutrients to the brain. The lung system controls qi intake and is also related to the brain. As you can see, all of the organs are in fact related to the brain. By exercising the brain, you help the body, and by exercising the body, you help the brain.

Working with qi is like working with an electric power plant. We use the electricity generated by the power plant to perform all kinds of functions. By elevating body energy with taiji or qigong, we can stimulate the brain and affect the brain chemicals. This kind of practice engages your attention, puts you into a state of calm, and raises your relaxation response. For centuries, Eastern philosophers have known the connection between our minds and our bodies; this is the basis of qigong.

All three components of qi practice—mental focus, body movement, and breath—affect our brain. A focused mind allows the brain to more easily carry out its functions, such as memorizing. Body movements, together with deep breathing, help energy go through the body smoothly, finally reaching and passing through the brain. As deep breathing is stimulating the respiratory and circulatory centers in the brain, it also gathers our attention. The body becomes like a well-tuned, biological supercomputer, as the network and the electricity reach equilibrium.

With the taiji workout, your energy starts moving in the body smoothly, your energy pathways are opened, your internal organs start to work harmoniously, and your mind and body start to work together. You are more adept, more open to learning, more willing to try new things and gain new experiences, and your brain cells start to communicate. New experiences create more connections among brain cells. This harmonious energy also promotes rapid healing.

8. Balancing the Emotions

Both the right and the left frontal lobes are very important for the regulation of emotion. They are needed for making decisions in both the social and personal realms. Because taiji stimulates the whole brain, coordinating the left and right brain and stimulating the crisscrossing of information between the left and the right brains and between the upper and lower brains, it also balances the limbic system, the emotion center. Neurotransmitters start flowing smoothly between the synapses. After seeing the changes in the emotional state of many of my students, I was compelled to write *Tai Chi for Depression* (YMAA, 2017).

Taiji balances emotion also by developing self-awareness, focus, and positive thinking, as well as by building strong qi. Emotional balance is very important for preventing brain aging and helps to provide the right mind-set for learning. Having balanced emotions enables you to be focused and pay attention to what you are doing. This helps both learning and memory. An impaired emotional state can reduce learning ability and make a person prone to memory loss.

Many people use medication to treat emotional problems. I disagree with this approach. They don't realize that many medications can cause memory loss, brain fog, and brain aging. A friend of mine, Lisa, a very sweet and intelligent person, is dealing with an emotional issue. She has been suffering from depression for a long time and is using medications. She has a hard time remembering things, especially appointments and dates.

9. Involvement in Martial Arts

We all know that martial arts practice is intended to make you strong and disciplined. Martial arts can give you mental power that helps you achieve. In almost every form of taiji, there is some martial arts relevance. People choose to practice taiji for different reasons: to find inner peace, for stress relief, for flexibility, for healing, for longevity, for increasing energy and stamina, or for competition and self-defense. Taiji originated as a martial art, and some movements are more pronounced in their martial aspect and can be used for self-defense. These martial arts movements make you feel stronger, more powerful, and more in control of yourself. They give you a solid, safe, stable, and determined feeling. They make you feel good and help you believe in yourself, which helps you succeed in anything you want to do. Whatever you do, you need to feel good about yourself. You cannot succeed if you don't feel good about yourself.

10. Adding the Right Music

Music is everywhere. We listen to music when we drive, walk, work out in the gym, sit in the doctor's or dentist's waiting room, or just relax at home. Music is important in our lives. Different music has different effects on people. Certain music can have healing effects. Soothing music harmonizes the brain, bringing about feelings of peacefulness. Loud, fast, heavy, driving music, on the other hand, can overstimulate the adrenal glands and brain, causing the release of noradrenaline and adrenaline, which increase heart rate and can create tension. All this can have negative effects on our heart, mind, and blood pressure. Long-term overstimulation can contribute to difficulty sleeping, interfere with immune function, and provoke attention deficit hyperactivity disorder–like behavior (as in not being able to handle quiet). Other kinds of music can make you depressed, sad, or anxious. Science has demonstrated the effects of music on our brains and on our health. Many studies have even shown that certain music can reduce tension and enhance specific types of intelligence, such as verbal ability and spatial-temporal reasoning.

In general, the music used in taiji practice is relaxing, gentle, calming, and tranquil. Adding music to taiji and qigong practice gives double benefits for well-being. Using relaxing music helps you slow the movements down and become more aware of your movement, relaxation, and feeling of unity. If you try to use different music, the results of practice may be different.

11. Responding to Relaxation

I have treated numerous patients who were loaded with stress. I cannot say that I don't have any stress, but I can say that taiji and qigong help me to manage it well most of the time. In addition, it helps me remain focused on what I am doing. Too much stress causes less blood flow to your muscles, which weakens the muscles (this can be proven with muscle-testing techniques). You then feel tired; even your brain feels tired. You may recall a time when you were stressed and could not think straight.

When you carry stress for long periods, eventually your muscles will degenerate, and you will feel pain all over your body. Your doctor then might give you a diagnosis called fibromyalgia. You may think that's the answer and a cure is sure to follow, but you do not have the answer. You only have a name that doesn't mean anything. If I were to give the condition a name, it would be "poor circulation, chronic inflammation, and degeneration in the muscle tissue." I have treated many people with "fibromyalgia." These people take many medications or painkillers but still have pain. Many of them develop other problems from the side effects of their medications. We now understand that to help fibromyalgia, the first thing is to get your blood and energy moving.

There are many ailments related to stress or tension over a long time, such as insomnia, headache, heart disease, hypertension, cholesterol, gastrointestinal problems, sexual dysfunction, back problems, neck problems, and inability to focus. In addition, stress causes distraction. You lose focus, and you lose your normal sense of what life is supposed to be like.

Taiji and qigong are meditation in motion, the best analgesic for all these symptoms. You relax, and all stress starts to melt away. Your body holds less tension; you feel calmer and more peaceful. The relaxation you get from taiji or qigong practice allows your energy to move smoothly through the body. Your overwhelmed brain gets a rest, your muscles relax, your emotions settle down, and the tiredness disappears. Your yin-yang energy flow and balance are restored. Once your muscles are relaxed, more blood flows to the muscle tissue. For this reason, your muscles become strong. You become more comfortable in your own skin, more aware of yourself in space and on the planet, and consequently more aware of where you hold the tension or feel the weakness. Now you've got something tangible to work on, which restores your sense of what life is supposed to be. Once you are more relaxed, you become more positive, and a positive state of mind can cause brain structure and function to change for the better. Your neurotransmitter levels become balanced, which is key to maintaining mood and emotion. This positive cycle gives you a balanced life and better health.

12. Becoming Rooted

With our modern lifestyle, we are distracted by so many activities and so much information. We don't know how to focus or what we are really attracted to. If you ask college students, even older ones, what they really want, many of them won't know how to answer. Some of them might just go for whatever job they can find to make a living, and others may be after a high-paying job. But what if it turns out that they are not happy with the money-making job?

Taiji and qigong help you feel rooted, stable, and focused, allowing you to find your passion. This kind of practice helps you become more aware of yourself and your spirit. It makes you more able to listen to your heart and soul. Taiji brings you closer to nature; it helps you think and act more naturally, more authentically. The more natural you are, the more you understand universal energy and how it works. Doing things in a natural way is part of the brain's learning pattern, and getting away from technology sometimes can bring great benefits. We eventually find what we truly want, what we are attracted to, what we do best, and what makes us happy. When you do a job you feel good about, the feeling is priceless. There is a saying: "Less is more." Being in tune with nature, you cannot go wrong.

13. Touching

Sometimes we rub sore muscles when we feel discomfort. Sometimes we massage our temples when we get headaches. If we fall and hurt a leg, we use our hands to press on the injured area. If you go to the doctor and tell her you have knee pain, within a few minutes, the doctor is offering to give you a prescription for your pain without even touching your knee. How does that make you feel? If your child has a headache, the first thing you do is to touch his head to feel if he has fever. You then rub his head, trying to make him feel better. Why is that? It is because touching is an important part of healing. Why do we need hugs and kisses? Because the sensation we get from them indicate friendship, love, and closeness. Affection creates the feeling of being cared for.

Touching can bring many benefits to our body, mind, and brain. Neuroscientists can see the effect of touch on the brain using functional magnetic resonance imaging. There is an increase in blood flow that is correlated with an increase in neuronal activity. Touch appears to affect multiple brain regions at both the conscious and unconscious levels. Touch has a wide range of impacts on the brain, influencing our sensations, movements, thought processes, and capacity to learn new movements.

Some of the warm-up exercises for taiji, and qigong itself, involve self-massage and acupressure. Through these kinds of sensory stimulation, not only do our brains get immediate benefit, but also our total awareness is heightened. Our bodies' acupressure points are stations on the energy map. You are delivering qi to these stations during self-massage and with slow, rhythmic breathing.

14. Group Energy

One of the best aspects of taiji and qigong are that they are not only ways to exercise but also make for a nice group activity. We are social beings. We seek others like ourselves to do the things we enjoy, to enrich our lives and spirit. Social activity brings a learning experience with it; the more you interact with people, the more you learn. Animals are the same—a dog loves to be part of a pack. Scientists are finding from animal study that animals raised in an enriched environment had at least twice as many new brain cells in the region of memory and learning as the control group. The stimulation of their environment also provoked the development of new connections (synapses) *between* neurons. They also found that animals that live in an enriched environment live longer as well.

Scientific research has repeatedly proven that social deprivation has severe negative effects on overall cognitive ability. Not only that, social deprivation can cause depression, anxiety, and other serious illness. For many people, daily exercise involves each individual working by themselves, either on the treadmill or elliptical machine, weight lifting, or running. We really don't have to interact with anyone else. In the gym, we usually work on individual groups of muscles, to speed our heart rate, to raise our blood pressure, work up a sweat to get our metabolisms going in hopes of losing some weight, gaining some muscle mass, and bringing more blood to our brain.

With taiji and qigong, it is different. It is recommended that they be done in a group (even though you sometimes need to practice by yourself). Group energy is important and very beneficial in taiji and qigong. Taiji in particular depends on a great deal of group energy, whether practicing in a classroom or outdoors. Group practice fosters discussion, friendship, social connection, group harmony, and all the positive benefits you might expect from group energy. Taiji and qigong also bring blood and oxygen to the brain and stimulate the connections between brain cells. The combination of practice and group energy can only enhance these effects. It is no wonder these arts are so helpful in preventing memory loss and enhancing learning ability. People who participate in group taiji class at our school feel happy, joyful, comfortable, and relaxed.

Students tend to do better when they practice together because the energy of each individual affects the energy of others in the class. The more energy channels an individual is able to open, the better the results will be from practice. When everyone's energy channels are open, the whole area is loaded with energy. You cannot see this, but you can feel it. In any kind of work, teamwork always brings the best results. The harmonious group energy makes you feel good for a long time afterward too.

This is what one of our participants said:

As a young man, I am capable of running a marathon and riding my bicycle one hundred miles. After I ran the Boston Marathon, I felt I had made my way to the top of the mountain: I did something that most people will never be able to physically do, for whatever reasons those may be. But even though I was in good physical shape, after starting my journey with taiji, I realized I had trouble coordinating my body in certain ways.

Since that short time ago and with much dedicated practice, I have improved my coordination tremendously. And I have humbly realized I am not at the top of the mountain but only at the beginning of a path!

Taiji has not only helped me physically but mentally and spiritually as well. I have been stuck in a dead-end retail environment for the past six years. Through the influence of coming to taiji and qigong classes, I am now going to school to be a holistic health counselor. . . . I believe my journey in taiji so far has empowered me to utilize a part of myself that was just lying dormant.

Therefore, even as a young man, I can personally attest to the all-encompassing well-being benefits of this awesome exercise!

—Matt G.

Other Tips for Brain Antiaging and Enhancing Learning Ability

Exercise

Physical exercise and body movement are crucial. It doesn't matter what kind of exercise you start with, Eastern or Western (though doing both is even better). Power walking is a great brain-fitness exercise. Walking with a friend and talking is very good for the brain because it adds that all-important social aspect. In a word, you just have to move your body. Qigong is a great exercise to start with because it is low impact, has little risk of injury, and works the whole body. My favorite exercise is therapeutic qigong (see my book *Natural Healing with Qigong*) (YMAA, 2004).

Keep Learning

Always try to think about ways you can improve yourself in all dimensions. You can learn a new language or learn to play chess or cards. You could take up knitting or even the piano, make things with your hands, become skilled at fixing things, learn a musical instrument, join a new organization, meet new people, and explore new places to vacation.

Read

We always tell kids to read more for their intellectual development. As adults, we should do the same thing. My father always admonished me when I did not read the newspaper when I was young. To please him, I started to read it. He was right: by reading the newspaper, I did learn a lot. Reading is always good for our brains. Reading aloud is even better because you also get brain stimulation from the sound.

Memorize Numbers

Practice remembering different number sequences—phone numbers, house numbers, birthdays, anything with a number. If you don't remember your Social Security number by now, you are in trouble. You will have to watch out for dementia or Alzheimer's disease later in life. If you don't have a memory problem now, that doesn't mean you don't need to practice memorizing number sequences. The more you practice, the better it is for your brain's health. Start practicing right away, and work on it every day. As the saying goes, "Use it or lose it."

Party and Socialize

As we discussed before, socializing is a type of learning experience and a great brain exercise. It definitely enhances your brainpower and promotes the connections of brain cells. Not only are you exposed to learning new things in a different way, but you are also encountering different personalities, levels of intelligence, information, backgrounds, cultures, food and drink, clothes, energy, and lots more. It makes a big difference in your life if you participate in social activities. I used to focus only on my work, feeling that going to social events was wasting my time. I was wrong because my old-timer training did not help my brain. I don't know if you have had this experience (I have encountered many people of this type): a great physician but pretty dumb in other ways, or a very smart scientist but with a poor lifestyle. Now that I do attend (and even host) social events, I find that I meet many different people and have made a lot of new friends. They are wonderful people to be with. Many of my students become my friends too. Life is just so much more colorful, and even though my mind is busy, it is not busy just with work. Almost all centenarians studied by science have had a strong social life—they tend to be outgoing, easygoing, multitalented, and hardworking. What more evidence do you need?

Sing

Singing, either with a group or on your own, accompanied or unaccompanied—even doing karaoke—is an excellent brain exercise and qi practice. When you sing, there is a lot going on in your body and your brain: you have to remember the words and the melody, and you have to try to stay in tune. These multiple stimulations make more connections in your brain's nerve branches and synapses. Next, you need to take big breaths to sing and hold the sound. The deep breathing and sound vibration make a great qi practice. Sound has energy. The vibration and energy stimulate the brain like a wake-up call. Singing helps you to quickly move qi and build better stamina.

I suggest that you try this experiment when you are driving and feeling tired and sleepy: just sing out loud and see what happens. Suddenly, you feel awake and alert. You can keep your eyes open. That's because you are moving qi.

Too many of us are shy about singing in public. When we offered karaoke at our office party, most people said, "I don't sing" or even, "You don't want to hear me singing." I had to keep telling them, "This is just for fun; it's not a competition!" Some people were willing to try, but others would not even pick up the microphone. My singing used to bother my American husband. He was not a big karaoke fan. So I stopped singing for many years. After a while, I realized I could not sing well anymore and felt somewhat depressed—something was missing in my life. When I went to visit China, I found out what it was. I went singing with my friends at a karaoke room. All of them sang better than me—and I used to be the best one! It was then that I realized, *It is the vibrational energy I am missing*. So I decided to sing whenever I got the chance. I would sing for my own health and have more fun in my life at the same time. Now, after many years of partying with karaoke, even my husband has come to like it!

I suggest you start to sing, even if it's just in the car while you are driving—for fun, for energy, and for exercising your brain. You won't be sorry.

Be Present

Whatever you do, you should pay attention to it. Paying attention to what you are doing helps you achieve better results. It helps you avoid stress too. If you have ten things to do, you should start one thing, focus on it, and finish it; then you can start working on the next thing, focus on it, finish it, and so on. In this way, you will get much more accomplished. Any time you get distracted, you need to remind yourself to be present and pay attention to the task at hand. Ask yourself very often, "What am I doing now? Where is my mind now?" This way you are able to get your thoughts back on track. Pay attention to where you are, who is around you, what subject is being discussed, and what is the goal of the task at hand. This helps to keep your brain to function optimally.

Chinese Medicine for Brain Health

Traditional Chinese medicine (TCM) is a mind-body medicine, a whole-health medicine. The meridian system goes through all body parts, including the brain. By stimulating these energy pathways, the brain receives signals. It is like flipping a switch to make better connections between nerve cells. People have told me that they feel more alert and that their minds are clearer. With the appropriate tune-up, your neurochemicals become balanced, and this helps to prevent brain aging and memory loss. If you get periodic care with TCM, you will definitely have fewer physical and emotional complaints. In Chinese medicine, it is always "two for the price of one" because the practitioner always tries to treat all of your multiple ailments. This is unlike Western medicine, where we have to go to so many different specialists for what are really related ailments.

TCM offers a variety of treatment modalities that look at all your complaints as related—after all, your body is one whole, and your mind and body form a single whole. So your health should be treated as whole too.

Acupuncture

Your meridian system is a big computer network. Stimulating certain points opens up the channels and therefore balances the mind and emotions. Acupuncture is a great way to keep your energy pathways open. There are many points on your body related to your brain. Unblock the pathways and stimulate the brain: that is what helps to balance brain chemicals.

Tui Na (Chinese Massage)

Massage also gives sensory stimulation to the brain, as discussed previously in the touch section. Tui na is an excellent therapy to keep you happy and an ideal alternative to acupuncture if you are afraid of needles. Some people like tui na so much they use it regularly as preventive medicine care. Periodic tui na helps you remain physically and mentally relaxed and emotionally balanced. You feel that you're getting true care with healing energy from the practitioner's hands.

One of my patients asked me if I am able to help children with emotional and learning disabilities. She told me that her daughter Mandy, age fourteen, had Asperger's syndrome. Mandy was on heavy medication and suffered from depression, weight gain, inability to focus or do schoolwork, anxiety, and anger issues. She could read for only a few minutes, and she had major social issues. I explained how natural medicine can help this condition, but I did not promise anything. She decided to make an appointment for her daughter with me.

When Mandy came to see me the first time, she did not look at me when she talked. She adopted a tough demeanor but seemed very upset and anxious, fidgeting throughout the appointment. She had no faith in herself and thought she was stupid, fat, and that nobody liked her. I did a meridian examination of her body and found that her body had blockages in many areas. She argued with me, disagreeing with my recommendations.

I explained in a calm tone how she could be helped with natural medicine and exercise. Finally, she became more open to the treatment. I did a combination of tui na, acupressure, and some qigong massage. She became a lot calmer right after the treatment. I then taught her three exercises and some simple qigong, which were targeted to her symptoms. I asked her to make sure to do them at home and also gave her some other homework, including a change in diet and some mental exercises.

When she came for the second visit, she was a different person. She had done the homework I'd given her that first visit, and she had changed her diet. She looked much calmer and spoke to me with a sweet smile, agreeing with my recommendations. When I checked her body meridians, her blockages were much better.

After five visits, she had lost weight, could read for much longer, and was doing her homework by herself. She also said her depression was gone. The whole family was very happy with her progress. But I knew she still had longer to go. As I mentioned before, learning should never stop.

Another patient, Dorothy, was diagnosed with dementia. She often forgot names, didn't remember events from the day before, and could not recall some commonly used words. Her husband, Mark, was frustrated. They came to me, and Dorothy was under my care for several months. The treatments and exercises I prescribed for her made a big difference in her language and memory. Mark could not believe it. Loss of memory in the aging process is normal, but we can certainly decelerate this with natural therapy. From Dorothy's case, we know that anything is possible, including delaying the damage of early aging.

Two patients sent me these letters:

Dear Dr. Kuhn,

THANK YOU. I have just come home from a treatment today, and I just feel simply amazing. The massage and the acupuncture treatments made me feel like I had lost about ten pounds, and I hit the gym after and had the best workout I've had in about a year. No pain in my knees or shoulders when I lifted or used the elliptical. So, thank you, thank you, thank you—and so far, I have called a few more of my friends and will hopefully be bringing them with me to see just how WONDERFUL you are.

—Anna H., Cape Cod, Massachusetts

Dear Dr. Kuhn,

I just wanted to share with you that I woke up this morning feeling alert and glad to be alive. (I don't often wake up that way.) I feel wonderful, have energy I haven't had in a long time, and best of all, have hope. Thank you so much. I love being alive again! All the best to you!

—Jennie K., New York

The Differences between Taiji and Qigong

"What is the difference between taiji and qigong?" This is a question I often hear from my students and people attending my workshops. In the United States, more people know about taiji than qigong. They don't associate the two. They see them as individual and separate Chinese exercises. In reality, both taiji and qigong are internal energy workouts. They are both a part of the same energy science. Taiji has a history of more than four hundred years, whereas qigong has a history of more than four thousand years. Qigong is clearly the father of taiji.

Taiji is a type of qigong, a higher-level qigong that requires many years to learn well. Taiji requires motor skill and coordination. Qigong requires no particular skill. Generally speaking, taiji is much more challenging, a deeper workout, and ultimately, more fun than qigong. There are five main styles of taiji: Yang, Chen, Wu/Hao, Wu, and Sun. They look different from each other when performed, but they are all based on the same basic principle. Chen style is the oldest, and Yang style is the easiest. The most popular styles in China and the United States are the easier Yang style followed by the Wu style and then the Chen style. The most powerful and the closest to martial arts is, first, the Chen style and then the Wu style. Besides being the oldest, Chen style is the most difficult form. All the taiji forms are, in some ways, a qigong workout.

Qigong is easier than taiji. It also has many different forms from which to choose. Some of them can be more difficult than others. Some people think qigong is too boring and not challenging enough. This is because they don't really know qigong well and haven't practiced it properly. If you practice qigong right, it is not boring at all.

Some qigong is a purely sitting meditation meant to purify the mind. Some forms of qigong work only on your body, while other forms work on both mind and body.

You should not need to separate these two exercises. Rather, think of them as brother and sister. I sometimes use qigong as a warm-up before taiji practice, and most students love it. I sometimes use taiji movements while practicing qigong, so that my students can feel the qi in their bodies and hands. Taiji practitioners who also practice qigong will sense qi sooner and learn taiji more quickly and easily.

If you are a beginner, I suggest you practice qigong first, then start to learn taiji after you feel the benefits of qigong. This way, you will know that qi does exist and can

Taiji	Qigong
Advanced energy workout	Beginner energy workout
Needs full concentration to achieve full benefits	Needs full concentration to achieve full benefits
Movements are slow and circular, slow paced with particular form and specific steps. Learning the sequence may initially be difficult. It takes a long time to learn a complete routine or form and takes even longer to master it.	Movements are simple, easy to follow, and easy to learn. Some forms can be repetitive. Foot placement is easy.
Movement only	Some qigong involves self-massage.
Five main styles or forms: Yang, Chen, Wu/Hao, Wu, Sun, and some variations	Five categories but more than a hundred forms: Daoist, Buddhist, Confucian, martial arts, and therapeutic
Breathing is slow and deep, coordinated with each movement.	Breathing can be slow or fast. It varies in different forms of qigong.
Related to martial arts	Related to natural medicine
Mostly practiced in walking motion	Can be practiced in any position but is mostly practiced in a standing position
Not practical for severe illness	Good for all kinds of illness; no restrictions
Beginners may be easily frustrated.	Some people may find it too simple.
Strong and solid results but may be long term	Immediate results, though long-term practice provides better results
Serves as a means of self-discipline	Serves as a means of self-therapy
Participants can be younger, but it is for all ages.	Participants can be older, but it is for all ages and all ability levels.

be felt. But you should not feel restricted. You may start to practice taiji anytime if you wish, as long as you understand that it is a long journey.

Both taiji and qigong can be used to heal the body and mind, nurture the spirit, strengthen internal energy, boost the immune system, and help you focus. Both can be your lifetime friends. Just keep in mind the differences listed in the table below.

Please Note: The above is a rough comparison, drawn from my own experience. But things are never really so black and white. This characterization of taiji and qigong is not meant to be rigid. You should experience each type of exercise for yourself in order to really understand its benefits. You might discover something different and more valuable in one or the other. Everything has multiple aspects. Some aspects are good for one person and other aspects are good for someone else. Some exercises may be right for me, and other exercises may be right for you. Try them and feel the differences. Find out for yourself what you enjoy about each of them. After you practice for a while, you may be surprised to discover something beneficial that other people may not have noticed.

Chapter 4

The Way to Wise Living

Commonsense Practice

COMMON SENSE MEANS "common knowledge everyone should have." But unfortunately, many people today don't seem to have it. Why is this?

We live in a dynamic world. Modern people are dynamic, and the flow of information is dynamic. We all assume we are smart and do things in a smart way. But we often lose our common sense to distraction, stress, illness or physical ailments, and emotional distress. Our focus is often on others—their successes, problems, and points of view. We often forget to pay attention to ourselves. This causes us to lose common sense.

Common sense is listening and paying attention to ourselves and to our world. It is considering what is going on with our health and the direction our lives are headed. What makes health fail? What makes our lives successful? Common sense involves knowing how to correct mistakes, make improvements, and assess our energy flow. *Am I balanced or imbalanced? What do I need to change to restore balance?* The bottom line is, we need to know how to make energy flow better, our lives flow better, and our work flow better by paying attention to ourselves.

There are a thousand different ways to get to your goals. By following your common sense, you will get there sooner. Some people regard me as wise. I cannot say I am wise, but I do follow my common sense. I observe, pay attention, and catch myself when I falter. I am open to insights outside my own field of expertise. I am willing to correct myself and change. If one way doesn't work, I go another way. If one method doesn't work, I use another. If a person makes me anxious, I choose to walk away and let him go his way. If a drug or herb cannot help me, I use exercise and diet instead. If I realize my memory is getting worse, I do things to improve it. And so it goes. In both my practice and my life, I have found that to go with the flow is better than to go against it.

Following common sense can help you in many ways. It can help you to relieve stress, do things more effectively, and find the right path.

A patient named Marianne came to see me for an initial visit. Just by looking at her, I asked myself, *What the heck has this girl been through?* She seemed incredibly stressed, looking much older than she actually was. Her hands were shaking, and her shoulders were drawn up and tight. The first thing I said to her was, "Can you put your shoulders down?" She replied, "I didn't know my shoulders were up." She then dropped her shoulders and laughed at herself. I then asked her to relax and convinced her that nothing would go wrong here.

After collecting her information and examining her body's meridian pathways, I realized that most of her problems were from her worry, anxiety, and fear. These created blockages in the energy pathways in her body, causing poor circulation, inflammation, and degeneration. Her heart, kidneys, spleen, liver, and lungs in the meridian pathways all had blockages, and so did all the organs they were associated with (which is not always the case). She had arrhythmia, a bladder problem, a bowel problem, indigestion, anxiety, depression, low energy, and back, neck, and shoulder pain. She had so many problems that it was no surprise she was depressed. Helping her would be a challenge, I felt.

Fortunately, I am not afraid of challenges. I always learn a lot from them, gain more experience, come away feeling that anything is possible, and am made stronger. I do have many challenged patients. Some are challenged by their attitude, others by their physical ailments. I did not limit Marianne's treatment to addressing physical problems or to unblocking her energy merely to promote circulation in her body. I also spent time helping her relax both her body and her mind, educating her with Daoism, and teaching her simple qigong exercises. I acted as a guide for her to find her own power and wisdom. Everyone has power, but not everyone knows it, and still others don't know how to use it. I merely opened a door for her and taught her to find her own power and how to use it. After six months, she was 90 percent better. A year later, she was a totally different person.

Another patient named Mark I worked with recently had an illness that was not getting better with treatment by his physician. He came to see me with many puzzle pieces. He was also very skeptical and anxious. He was straightforward when he said, "Americans don't want to change. We don't believe anything else but 'go to doctors, use whatever doctors give us, and accept whatever procedures they want us to undergo.' We like to do things fast and get the quick fix—just get it done. We don't want to wait.

We worry about everything—job, kids, retirement, security, career. . . ." Finally I had to say to him, "That is why you have heart disease."

In Chinese medicine, the heart is related to the mind and thought processes. An overwhelmed mind affects your heart and heart energy. This could lead to insomnia, anxiety, loss of focus, forgetfulness, poor circulation, or—like my patient—heart disease. I not only had to use Chinese medicine to help his heart, but I also had to educate him. I taught him techniques for balancing his heart energy and to relax. This is a long journey but one well worth traveling.

We always say, "Good things take time." Don't get discouraged if you fail several times as you try to put theory into practice. You will have many opportunities to get back on track and be successful. Important undertakings take time. Time allows you to learn, heal, forgive others, use common sense instead of emotion, and allow you to find what really makes you happy. We should not waste time but use it wisely because it is so valuable. Time is like a river. It flows in only one direction.

In his book *The Tao of Power: Lao Tzu's Classic Guide to Leadership, Influence, and Excellence*—a translation of the *Dao De Jing*—R. L. Wing writes,

> *The brain accepts all types of information from all stimuli simultaneously, and the mind processes it in the form of emotional responses, intuitive feelings, and logically formulated analyses. In the West, we rely almost exclusively on logical analysis. We are encouraged to think in a linear fashion, using words and numbers to draw conclusions about our work and our lives. These logical functions, according to neurological research, are performed by the left hemisphere of the brain. At the same time, we learn to discount aesthetic or intuitive information—a right hemisphere function—because it is considered less valuable to our culture. Thus we find ourselves primarily concerned with measuring events and analyzing their meaning, rather than creating and directing their flow. We are taught to ignore the intuitive or irrational, no matter how strong these "gut feelings" might be. As these right hemisphere feelings are repressed, we lose touch with our intuitive mind, and our insights become increasingly rare.[6]*

6. R. L. Wing, *The Tao of Power: Lao Tzu's Classic Guide to Leadership, Influence, and Excellence* (New York: Doubleday, 1986), 15.

The Secrets to Happiness

Happiness helps our brains and bodies maintain balance, and it prevents brain and body aging. You can see a person aging fast if she is not happy. Everyone deserves happiness, but not everyone knows how to find it. It cannot be found in external place, another person, or another job. It is from you. *You make happiness happen.*

When you are not happy, there are three things that may need to be addressed. Your mind may be troubled, tangled, or disturbed by negativities that bring your spirit low. The energy in your body may be blocked, stagnant, or not flowing properly. You may have lost direction in your life. When a person is happy, the mind is clear and healthy. The body's energy is harmonized and flows smoothly. Here are some good ways to bring an overall sense of happiness to your life.

1. Exercise Regularly

Many people try to eat well to restore their health. Many publications emphasize dieting and nutrition. Eating well is absolutely important, but diet is not enough. I have many patients who spend lots of money on supplements but still do not feel well. The parts of the body are either made for movement or involve movement: joints, muscles, organs, tissues, and all the rest. We have to move in order to stay healthy. In my experience, exercise is more important than diet alone.

There are both Western and Eastern forms of exercise you can choose. Jogging, walking, running, swimming, tennis, hiking, taiji, qigong, martial arts, and aerobic exercises are all beneficial to our brains. The bottom line is that you have to move your body.

2. Keep a Positive Attitude

Our brains have such power to control our lives. The brain controls the mind, the mind controls behavior, and behavior is the vehicle that drives life in many different directions. Our brains and minds can make all the difference in life. They can make our lives miserable or make our lives joyful. They can destroy us and others. They can bring a lifetime of happiness and success. There is a Daoist story about different mind-sets.

Three men were walking down the road. They were passing a corner and saw a spider climbing the wall. Because the wall in that area was wet, the little spider fell down. The little spider climbed up a second time, then fell again; it climbed and fell repeatedly. Watching the little spider made all three men think about their own lives.

The first man thought, "My life is like this little spider: climbing all my life and always falling."

The second man thought, "Look at that: life is full of mistakes. If we took a moment, we could find different ways to do things. This little spider could find another place to climb where the wall is dry; then it might reach the top of the wall."

The third man thought, "I am so affected by this little spider. It does not give up! Even after falling so many times, it continues to climb with seemingly unlimited energy. If I can do this, I am sure I can succeed."

This story shows that the direction our lives take can depend on our thoughts. Here's another Daoist story.

A man had traveled a long way after preparing for a long time to take a test to become a government officer. The night before the test, he had three dreams while staying in a hotel. The first dream was that he was planting vegetables on a high wall; the second dream was that he was holding an umbrella over his head while he wore a rain hat; the third dream was that he was asleep next to a woman he loved but back to back. He realized these three dreams were strange and needed to be interpreted and found a man who claimed he could interpret the dreams.

The man said to the dreamer, "Your life is dull; you plant vegetables on a wall, you are wasting your energy; you wear a rain hat, but you also carry an umbrella; you are doing useless work. You have a lover, but you are back to back sleeping on the bed; how can you make love?"

This man who had prepared for the test was very upset, depressed, and disappointed; he decided not to take the test. He gathered his luggage to go home. The hotel owner saw him packing, then asked him, "Why are you leaving for home? Aren't you supposed to take a test today?"

The man told the hotel owner about the three dreams and their interpretation. The hotel owner said to him, "I know how to interpret dreams too, and you had good dreams. The first dream tells you that your position will be high; the second dream tells you that you are assured to have total coverage; the third dream tells you it is time to turn around." The dreamer felt much more confident after he heard this explanation. He decided to go forward and take the officer test. He did very well too, and passed it. A year later, he got a good government job.

This story tells us that life is a test: you can move forward or you can quit, depending on your mind-set and how you think about things.

We live in a world with negatives and positives. If we focus on the negatives, it makes us vulnerable, stops us from moving forward, blocks our energy channels, and makes us feel down, debilitating us and making us feel old. As soon as we change our focus, life changes and the whole world changes.

Being positive is the way to success and happiness. If you have a positive attitude and take positive action, you most likely will be successful in whatever you do. If you fail, you can always get up and start over again; failure can teach us what doesn't work. Failing is a part of life's journey; there is no such thing as never failing.

When you have a positive attitude, people like to be with you. They become cheerful, and they feel good when you are around. Not many people like to be with someone who is negative. You lose friends that way. When you have no friends, depression becomes more pronounced. It is like a negative circle: everything becomes worse and worse. Without a change in attitude or a change in your way of thinking, even antidepressants are less likely to be helpful.

A former patient of mine had clinical depression. His main problem was negativity. He could not see the positive side of things, and we know that everything has two sides. He lost friends one after the other, and he lost girlfriends one after the other. He continued to feel lonely, frustrated, powerless, and hopeless. He had no energy and no job. Complaining about his illness all the time, he blamed his doctor for being unable to help him. He felt he was unable to work. He refused to do qigong, taiji, or any other exercise. He complained that his medications had many side effects, but he wanted to continue to use them. He sank further and further into the darkness, feeling depressed even though he went to a therapist on a weekly basis. This kind of person is very difficult to treat because he does not have a positive attitude and is not willing to change his way of thinking. He would not let go of the negativity in his life and get better.

3. Don't Be Afraid of Hard Work

People have told me many times, "You work hard." Yes, I work very hard and learn very hard, too. Living in two different countries, each of which has undergone many changes, there is so much to learn. Hard work can be a good learning experience. Some people complain that they work too hard. If you don't enjoy what you are doing, the complaint is reasonable. However, many studies tell us that over 90 percent of healthy older people worked hard in their lifetimes and volunteered in later life as well. If you enjoy the work you do, even if it is hard work, it can still be rewarding. If you complain about everything you do, you are in trouble, and it is wise to seek help. Complaining creates negative energy that not only makes you unhappy but affects other people as well. You should look for enjoyment in working with different people, encountering new knowledge, and getting paid for your hard work.

4. Be Honest with Yourself and Others

Honesty is an important part of living in harmony. The world would be a different place if we were all honest. Honesty creates trust, trust creates harmony, and harmony leads to happiness. Loss of trust in family, friends, business associates, or politicians creates problems in our lives and in society. Losing trust does not bring good results.

Many of my patients have said to me, "I have trust in you; I know you can help me." This kind of mind-set makes my work easier. It allows me to do my best and make the healing work more effective too. My father always told me, "Always be honest. You have nothing to lose." I grew up in an honest family. I studied medicine with an honest heart, and I do business in an honest manner. I treat patients with honesty. If I cannot help a patient, I tell the truth. This makes my life a lot easier and less stressful, and my patients appreciate being treated with respect.

Some people play mind games or manipulate for their own advantage. Or they fail to do what they really want to do because they are afraid of being criticized. This creates blockages. They don't understand that if they are honest, they have nothing to fear. Constant tension creates stress and blockages in your energy system and also makes your life tiring and stressful. You cannot be truly happy when you carry tension and stress.

5. Help Other People

Human beings have always helped one another in order to survive and live well. For example, in China, family members, friends, and coworkers all help one another to a degree that would be unusual in the West. Because of this, even in the past when they had lower incomes, the Chinese were considered a happy culture. That culture of happiness persists in most rural areas and provinces.

From many years of observation and experience, I have found that people who tend to give more are happier than people who tend to take more. When you help other people or give to people, you get a psychological reward. The positive action makes you feel good. If you think you lose something by helping others, or if you are worried that you are giving too much and not getting back, calculating whether it is fair or not fair, you create tension and stress that cause blockages in your body, in your mind, in your life, and in your relations, which affect your health. The calculation of "How much do I get?" weakens your spirit. Give for the sake of giving, and don't feel the need to get back. Giving is priceless if it is from your heart, and nothing can measure the value. You will be a lot happier because you will know you have something to offer. Life is about *creating* happiness, not getting it.

I sometimes do volunteer work for nonprofit organizations, even if I have to postpone my own work. Volunteering is not a waste of my time because I enjoy working with other people and learning new things too. I enjoy being productive and generous for something I believe in, and I enjoy the group energy. This has had a very positive impact on my spirit, and I have learned a lot from all kinds of group activity.

6. Avoid Overanalyzing

There are major differences between the Western and Daoist ways of processing things mentally. It is like left brain versus right brain. This is not about which one is better; it is about wisely using the wisdom of both because both Western and Eastern mental habits have strengths.

The Western mind analyzes everything, always trying to figure out why and how. But in some cases, when you try to analyze or insist on an exact answer, you end up overanalyzing and creating an ongoing battle within yourself. You may understand the cause of problems, but you may not know how to solve them. Things happen for many reasons and can be handled in many different ways.

The Daoist mind-set uses the Daoist philosophy to correct the imbalance in your mind, to help you let go of whatever is bothering you and thereby preserve your energy and your spirit. It is intuitive rather than logical. You follow your intuition and common sense rather than overanalyzing. You live with flow, or as we often say, "Whatever floats your boat." There is wisdom in this.

I had a patient named Jessica with many mental and emotional issues. She had been seeing a psychotherapist all her life but still had many problems. She was unable to let go of the past. She totally understood where her problems came from, but she could not make things better. She still blamed her parents for things that happened in her childhood. She held on to negative thoughts that caused worry and stopped her from participating in positive activities. She worried about things that would probably never happen, which was a complete waste of energy. Caution is good, but worry creates negativity that depletes your energy and creates blockages in your body's energy pathways. We don't need extra worry that troubles our health; our minds are already too busy from too much information. People think too much, worry too much, plan too much, and fear too much. This behavior creates stress and tension and can trigger depression, anxiety, and panic attacks.

The Dao teaches us to relax, to let go of negatives, to find balance and inner peace, to discover the power inside ourselves, to find our wisdom and let it guide our way to light. You cannot control or predict everything that happens. The more you analyze, the more problems you may have. I suggest you not waste energy this way but preserve it for more important things like improving health, happiness, and well-being. Find ways to deal with challenges practically and in the moment. If you adopt this way of thinking, I am sure you will see much improvement in your life.

7. Forgive Others; Forgive Yourself

"True forgiveness includes total acceptance. And out of acceptance, wounds are healed and happiness is possible again."

—Catherine Marshall

Forgiving others can create positive energy and help you to heal, let go, move on, and succeed. We all make mistakes in our lives, and we can all learn from them. Love can create forgiveness, and forgiveness can nurture love.

"Only the brave know how to forgive; it is the most refined and generous pitch of virtue that human nature can arrive at. A coward never forgives; it is not in his nature."

—Laurence Sterne

Some people tend to hold on to what is insignificant and negative. Letting go of unpleasant things that happened in your past can make your life easier. When you hold on to negative things, you lock yourself in a cage, and you have no freedom. Once you are able to let go, you set yourself free. Your energy channels are opened, your mind is free, and your happiness returns. Try to remember that every day is a new day, a new life. Life is like water constantly flowing with no end. It flows in one direction and does not flow back. We don't need to always bring back the old, especially what was not pleasant. When I talk about letting go of the old negative stories, some will argue with me, "We have to remember the past so we can learn from it." Yes, we can learn from the past, but this should be in the context of a transformation from negative to positive, a change for the better. Constantly remembering the negative parts of the past creates negative energy that misleads us and causes some degree of blockage in our emotions and mental processes. Then we don't really learn from the past. Remember, what is unpleasant is gone forever. So learn from the past by all means, but don't get stuck in negativity.

8. Use Daoist Wisdom in Everyday Life

I'll say it again: learning Daoist philosophy and living with Daoist wisdom can help you to become natural and spontaneous. You can then be more relaxed, accepting, tolerant, appreciative, and positive. Chinese people have used Daoism for centuries in almost every field. The military uses the Dao to make correct battle strategies. Scientists use the Dao to figure out how to make things happen. Chinese doctors use the Dao to help patients get well in the most efficient way. Teachers use the Dao to provide quality and balanced teaching. Astronauts use the Dao to stay focused on their mission. Farmers use Daoism to predict the weather and to prepare for planting and harvesting. The Chinese believe that if you use Daoist wisdom, you are more likely to succeed. Anyone can take advantage of this philosophy and use this ancient wisdom to help themselves. This wisdom does not directly tell you what to do, but it does give you a light to help you see things more clearly. It teaches you to unburden yourself, free your mind, and let things happen spontaneously and naturally. When you are really into Daoist practice, you are less likely to be affected by any kind of negativity.

Here is a Daoist story about Zhuang Zi, an influential fourth-century Chinese philosopher.

> A man asked Zhuang Zi, "You have been giving wisdom to others; your intelligence is superior—why is it you are not in a superior position?" Zhuang Zi replied, "The monkeys are playful in the big mountain; they can display their intelligence freely and nimbly. When they are in the jungle with so many thorns, they are helpless in moving their bodies and unable to display their skills. But as soon as they go back to the mountain, they can display their skills again."

The story tells us to be patient; we all have our own place to exhibit our skill.

Generally speaking, the natural way cannot go wrong. If you are against the natural way, you may be confronted with many obstacles. Through Daoist study and practice, you can be happy whether you are rich or poor, at any intellectual level, in any occupation, and at any age. Daoist practice can also accelerate healing. The bottom line is that you have to open your mind to all possibilities and let go of what is not helpful.

Again, from Wing's translation of the *Dao De Jing*:

> True power is the ability to influence and change the world while living a simple, intelligent, and experientially rich existence. Powerful individuals influence others with the force of example and attitude. Within groups, they have great presence—intellectual gravity—that influences the minds of those exposed to them. Intellectual gravity develops as a result of expanded identification—an identification that reaches far outside the self. Individuals who can identify with the evolution of reality develop significance and power because the force of their awareness is actively defining the universe around them. There are two major changes that occur in the lives of individuals who achieve personal power: the rise of intellectual independence and the need for simplicity. Daoism, as a way of understanding the universe, is not based on faith; it is based on experience. The human mind is evolving, while all social systems are temporary experiments. Relying on systems of understanding created or interpreted by others will

dull the instincts and prevent individuals from cultivating and expanding their own minds.[7]

9. Continue Learning, and Keep Your Mind Open

As we've discussed, lifelong learning is a crucial part of brain health and overall well-being. A closed mind is an obstacle to health and happiness. Often, people are taught in a certain way and pass on that way of thinking, generation after generation. Willingness to change goes together with a willingness to learn. Learning is an important part of making things change for the better. Open your mind, learn from many different sources, and learn from the past, but don't stay in the past. This will help you understand life better, see things from multiple angles, and make better decisions in all situations.

10. Cherish Love and Friendship in Your Life

"Love comes when we take the time to understand and care for another person."
—Janette Oke

We all have the ability to give love and experience the joy of being loved. Love can be interpreted in ways other than just the love between the romantically involved. Love between mother and daughter or son, friends, siblings, you and your pet, and you and your parents are examples of the many varieties of love. All love should be appreciated and cherished. There is an old saying in China: *Once you become a friend, you are a friend forever.* On one of my trips to China, a girl who has been my friend since middle school gave me a big punch as soon as she saw me. The reason she punched me was because I hadn't told her earlier I was coming to China. I had to apologize ten times while laughing hysterically. Sometimes people don't cherish friendships and may even abuse a friendship. Remember, if you give love, you also receive love. If you abuse friendships, you will never have true friends. Here is a rule of thumb: *If you don't like other people to treat you unpleasantly and with disrespect, you should not treat them that way.*

7. Wing, *The Tao of Power*, 13.

I believe that sharing love, being honest, forgiving, understanding, helping, caring, and giving to one another all help to avoid problems. If you always think about *me, my comfort, my pleasure, my life,* or *my needs*, without thinking much about the good of others, you will have difficulties in marriage and friendship. Love helps you understand better. With love, many problems can be solved.

"We can do no great thing, only small things with great love."

—Mother Teresa

Chapter 5

Get with the Program and Stay Young

WE HAVE DISCUSSED so much about the whys and hows of health and happiness. Now we need to put what we've learned into action. Without action, nothing can be achieved. A patient once told me, "I still have your qigong DVD from five years ago, but I haven't tried it yet." So, what are the benefits of purchasing my qigong DVD but never using it? Another person said to me, "I love your book. I am going to follow the advice you give in it as I try to lose weight." I asked him, "When are you going to start?" He answered, "I don't know yet." I would have preferred to hear him say, "Next month" or even "Next year." That would've been better than "I don't know yet," which may mean never.

Many people are thinkers. They think and think, but nothing gets done. Some people are doers, and even if they fail, they learn from the failure and improve. This is not to say thinking is unimportant; obviously it is. But I suggest you do both. Think about your goal, make a plan for attaining it, then follow that plan.

Learning Approach

There are two kinds of learning and practice: old-school learning and new-school learning. Old-school learning emphasizes the practice of basics and building a foundation before starting. In the Shaolin Temple's early years, students had to carry water to the mountain every day for a certain number of days before learning any martial arts skill.[8] Modern martial arts training often preserves emphasis on preliminary training: students may need to do many kicks, punches, jumps, splits, and running

---

8. The Shaolin Temple, a monastery in Henan Province, China, is the home of the martial arts school of gongfu (kung fu).

before learning martial arts forms. In learning taiji too, students traditionally need to practice "cat walk stance," shifting, turning, and qigong every day for many days before learning the form.

New-school learning focuses on form practice. Taiji skill is actually built on practicing the form. When one form is learned well, other forms are easier to learn.

Both schools of learning have advantages and disadvantages. Old-school learning is more difficult, boring, and may result in loss of students. But this kind of learning definitely allows the practitioner to build solid skills on the basis of a strong body and powerful core energy. And the skills transfer to self-defense. New-school learning is a little easier, more flexible, and the focus on form makes it more fun. It is good for the brain and promotes new connections in brain cells. But new-school learning doesn't give you fighting ability.

Because each individual has different needs, you can choose how you want to learn.

Fundamental Principles of Taiji Practice

For your study and practice to be effective, you need to understand taiji's principles.

Understanding the principles will make the learning process easier, and your taiji journey will be a whole lot easier too. A solid grasp of the principles also translates to better skills, more health benefits, better qi circulation, and better martial skill.

Taiji Mental Status and Physical Postures

When you start taiji practice, the first thing you need to learn is relaxation. This is easier said than done. In all the classes I have taught, I must have asked my students to relax a million times.

Your Mind

Your mind comes first in learning, healing, and antiaging. When practicing taiji or qigong, you need to *focus* on the body movements and energy center. Don't let your shen (mind and spirit in Chinese) walk away. You must focus solely on your own energy, and then you will see that it is possible to both perceive it and make it flow properly. When you understand that you are on the way to successful practice, you will practice without any hesitation.

Your mind's intention should be on taiji or qigong, your thoughts focused only on your body and relaxation. Once your mind is relaxed, your body becomes relaxed. If there is any tension, you need to get rid of it. Your eyes are not focused on any one object but take in your surroundings with full awareness. The mind produces *internal movement*, and internal movement produces *external movement*. All movements are directed from your mind. If your mind is not there, it will not be possible to work with your qi. Just as with anything else, if your mind is off track, you will not be able to do things successfully.

Your Shoulders

Your shoulders should be relaxed. Your elbows should be relaxed and about forty-five degrees from the body. Elevating your elbows or shoulders creates tension in your arms and shoulder area. From a martial arts standpoint, relaxing your shoulders and dropping your elbows is a protective strategy. If your shoulders are raised, your elbows will also be lifted. Then you are giving the opponent the chance to take you down or lock you up. Only if you are relaxed are you able to respond quickly to any movement by your opponent. Your arms should follow your body in every movement of taiji. You do not intentionally move the arms but let the arms go wherever the body goes. If you focus too much on your arm work, you look like you are dancing rather than doing taiji.

Your Wrists and Hands

Your wrist should be relaxed and flexible but well controlled. Relaxed doesn't mean floppy and having no strength, however, and controlled doesn't mean rigid. When your wrists are relaxed but not weak, you have the readiness you need if confronted with a fighting situation. Although taiji is not designed specifically for fighting, it serves as a self-defense tool as well.

Your hands should also be relaxed, with fingers slightly closed together.

Your Torso, Back, and Legs

Your torso and back should be relaxed. Relaxing your back allows for a smooth flow of energy. Your back carries the nerve system that directs all parts of your body. Keeping the back healthy is important in the prevention of many health problems. Back tension creates stagnation in the back meridians and the nerve system that is related to your whole organ system and body parts. No matter how you move your body, your back should be upright and relaxed. You will be very uncomfortable if your body is twisted or bent. You can get hurt or injured if you practice with an incorrect posture. You can tuck the buttocks inward to keep the lower back straight.

From a martial arts point of view, the waist, or abdomen, is your *powerhouse*. When your abdomen is loose, the power generated by your legs can be easily transmitted to your arms through your waist. Your waist can also generate power that directly moves energy to your hands. If your waist is stiff or tight, the power generated from your legs cannot be transmitted to your hands. Your powerhouse will therefore have less power. Ancient taiji masters stated, *The root is at your feet, power is initiated by your legs and directed by your abdomen, then expressed through your hands.*

Your knees should be bent during the entire taiji practice. You don't have to bend very low, however. For beginners or seniors, you can just unlock your knees. Advanced students or younger people with a flexible body and strong legs can bend the knees a little lower. It depends on the individual's ability. Doing it correctly is more important than maintaining a low stance. With each shifting of weight and turning of the waist, you can clearly distinguish between substantial (full) and insubstantial (empty) yin and yang movement. A simple way to grasp the meaning of substantial or full is to put all or most of your weight on one leg—that leg is now "substantial" or "full." Your other leg with little or no weight on it is "insubstantial" or "empty." Once you begin to understand the idea of substantial and insubstantial, you will have a centered and balanced feeling and be solid and grounded no matter what the movements may be. If you do not feel balanced, that means you just need to practice more.

Once you have relaxed all parts of the body, your entire body should be rooted, balanced, and centered, just like a tree. The strong roots of a tree can withstand a heavy wind or storm. Once the entire body relaxes, you will feel your internal "generator" is in standby mode, ready to generate energy. This is a very important skill to learn in taiji practice. It also helps you relieve stress, detach from all the junk in your mind, and let go of all tensions.

Taiji is a whole-body exercise that involves coordination of all body parts. Through taiji practice, you will improve your coordination too. One taiji principle from an ancient master states, *When there is an upward movement, then there is also a downward movement; when there is a left movement, then there is also a right movement.* Your body moves before your arm; your leg moves before your body. Each part of the body follows, one after the other.

Your Breath

Breathing is important in both taiji and qigong practice. Breathing should be deep, slow, and coordinated with the movements. In taiji practice, the breath should be fully addressed with advanced students but not with beginners because it can cause confusion due to the complexity of coordinating breath with the already-complex taiji movements. As you practice for a while and master the whole form, you can start to pay more attention to your breathing. Generally speaking, you breathe out when you direct energy out, and you breathe in when you bring energy in. Certain movements have different breath patterns that you will learn eventually. Some breathing techniques in qigong can be confusing, especially if you have never learned *how to breathe correctly* before. But you will learn from your instructor. You should not be afraid to ask your instructor about breathing, difficult movements, or any other questions at all.

Taiji Basic Movement Requirements

As we've said, taiji is a whole-body exercise. Whenever there is movement, the whole body moves. When one part of your body moves, all other parts also move. There is motion in stillness, and there is stillness in motion in every movement. We've noted the saying of the ancient taiji masters that movements are rooted in the feet, initiated from the leg, controlled by the waist, and shaped by the hands and fingers. Being rooted in your feet creates the strong roots of the tree, and then your legs start to move, followed by the waist. This is how the sequence appears in movement.

The upper and lower parts of the body are coordinated; left and right are coordinated; mind and body are coordinated; breathing and movements are coordinated. Do not worry if you have poor coordination. It will improve with practice. All movements are in a circular and continuous motion. There are many things in the natural and physical world that are in the shape of a circle, such as the earth and other heavenly bodies, their motion through the heavens, the eye, and many fruits and vegetables. Even electricity flow has to be a complete circuit with no breaks. Many of the circles have energy. This is part of the reason why the circular motion is so important in taiji practice.

Your weight is continually shifting from left to right and then from right to left. The waist position is also constant and continues turning from side to side. This describes the yin and yang of taiji movements.

Taiji Practice Requirements

Have Discipline

Developing taiji discipline is very important to your practice. It takes effort and mind power. You have to constantly remind yourself that you are a special person, that your hard work will pay off, and that you are not wasting your time. Discipline can take you to the place you want to be and lead you to your goal.

Be Patient

Nothing worthwhile comes easily or overnight. Feeling frustrated only gets you down and makes you sick. Taiji is a natural healing practice, and what is natural sometimes takes time. There is no shortcut or quick way to learn. If you don't get it right this week, maybe you will next week, or next month, or next year. It doesn't matter how long it takes. Many people think that learning the form is all there is to taiji. But learning the taiji form is not the whole story. To learn it correctly may be difficult and may take a long time. But if you want to see the beauty of a mountain view, you have to plan a trip and hike to the top. This can be hard work, but the payoff is the view. Many taiji masters in China have studied for a lifetime and still practice regularly.

In Chinese martial arts, there is no belt awarded. The reward is inside the practitioner. It is in combat that you see the practitioner's real level of attainment. People look for shortcuts to success, but shortcuts don't allow you to build a solid foundation of knowledge and skill. Only a solid foundation built through hard work can serve as a platform for success.

Have Confidence

I have often seen the effects of a lack of confidence. Confidence and pride are two different things. People who have too much pride may not have enough confidence.

Pride has to do with externals while confidence comes from within, from your mind and the way you think. Worry, fear, and laziness can diminish your confidence.

Everyone has strengths and weaknesses; there is no such thing as perfect. What is easy for one person to learn may be difficult for someone else. However, everyone can learn if they choose to, are determined, and if they put their minds to it. You might feel discouraged when you first begin taiji, but once you practice for a while, your confidence will build.

Practice with Diligence

Without diligent practice, you will not develop your taiji skill, and you will not reach your goal. Compare a doctor who just graduated from medical school and a doctor who has practiced for twenty years. Whom would you choose? This is just a simple example. If you need service from a company, would you choose a new company or a well-known one that has been providing the service for many years? Remember, good skill comes from diligent practice. The practice of taiji or qigong should be fun and not a chore. If you think it is fun, you will practice regularly. And group practice makes diligent practice a party.

Be Noncompetitive

There is no competition in taiji. There is no need to compare your skill to other people's skills. Taiji is for health maintenance, disease prevention, the healing of illness, as well as for building inner peace and delaying aging. Don't worry if someone else's coordination seems better than yours. So what? Watch and learn. You compete with only yourself to improve day to day. In many martial arts, you earn belts of different colors as you progress toward mastery. Taiji is different. There are no belts in taiji practice. What counts is how much you have improved over time—in relaxation, coordination, physical health, emotional health, mental alertness, creativity, learning ability, relationships, and overall quality of life.

Always Warm Up before Training and Cool Down After

It is important to do warm-up exercises before practice and to cool down after practice. I strongly recommended doing the warm-up exercises described in this book because they are designed specifically to stimulate your brain. You may choose any of these exercises. I designed them to help get your qi and blood flowing well through your whole body and to loosen your muscles and joints. They help to balance your emotions, enhance your brain-cell communication, and promote organ harmony. In addition, they speed heart rate and promote circulation, which is another benefit to the brain and aid in the prevention of brain aging. If you prefer, however, you could also use power walking or jogging for a warm-up.

After practice, you should not immediately become inactive. You should let your muscles slowly cool down with the cool-down exercises in this book. Muscles suddenly going from warm to cool cause stagnation of the blood circulation, muscle stiffness, and an increase in the possibility of muscle and tendon problems in the future. Many athletes experience muscle stiffness and inflammation of the soft tissue due to improper cool-down.

Practice Frequently

People often claim, "I don't have time today to practice." But it is not about whether you have time. You might *never* have time. It is about whether you *make* time. This concerns priorities. If your priority is health, you will make time for health-related activities. If your priority is learning, you set aside time to study or practice. Whatever you choose to do with your time, however, you may not be able to do it if you lose your health.

In preventive medicine, we encourage people to put a priority on health. When you lose your health, you lose everything. To benefit from taiji and qigong, it is best to practice every day, even if it's just the warm-up exercises or at least some of them. At a minimum, set your intention to practice three to five times a week.

Don't feel bad if you miss practice once in a while. As long as you have the intention, you can make up for it at your next practice. You may find you feel it when you miss practice. That is a good sign. You will know you are doing something right. We call this a *healthy craving*.

These exercises are designed to meet specific needs. For instance, if you feel down, practice the exercise for emotional balance described in chapter 6. When time is limited, you can prioritize in this way.

Practice Outdoors

When practicing outdoors, avoid strong winds and extreme cold or hot temperatures. Strong wind and extreme cold distract your attention and affect energy flow around your body. It is difficult to achieve good circulation in cold weather. Extreme heat might cause dehydration or heat stroke.

You should avoid wearing a hat during your practice. When you are bending forward, your hat may fall off, and picking it up would be a distraction. There is an acupuncture point on the top of your head called the bai hui point, or "hundred convergences" point, on the governing vessel meridian. It receives energy from above and then connects to all other energy channels in the body. You want that point open as you practice these qi exercises.

Practice with a Group

As we discussed before, working with a group can generate better results. It is more fun too. Attending regular classes helps you learn good habits and correct routines. The positive social environment gives you positive feedback and reinforcement. If you cannot find a quality teacher, you can always start your own group. Following a video-tape or DVD to learn is adequate but more difficult. For learning taiji, I designed a sequence called Taiji Basics, which is great for beginners. It is the bridge to self-study of taiji in any form. Self-study of qigong is not difficult as you can do it just by following a DVD. But it is so much better if you can find a good instructor.

Practice with Your Opposite Side

If you already know a taiji form very well, you can start to practice "opposite side" or "mirror side." If an exercise normally begins with a movement to the left, say, you begin instead with a movement to the right when you practice opposite side. This definitely enhances the connection of brain cells. Practicing opposite side may be very different in the beginning, but it will get better with practice. You'll soon realize your overall ability is improving as well as your memory. If you want to focus on the martial arts aspect of taiji, it is ideal for you to do opposite-side practice to further stimulate both sides of your brain. You will get optimal benefits from this approach. If you are a beginner, this is a perfect way for you to exercise both sides of the brain.

Don't worry about how well you do. What matters is that you do it. Taiji practice has no judgment; you do it at your own pace and ability. You will benefit as long as you follow the guidelines and principles.

Much more information about taiji theory and practice can be found in my book *Natural Healing with Qigong* (YMAA, 2004).

Chapter 6

Brain Fitness Practice

BEFORE YOU START to practice, check yourself for tension, weakness, and energy level. Do you have fear or worries? How relaxed are you, and what is your stress level?

After this performing this self-assessment, you are ready to begin practice, which has four steps. Begin with the total-body warm-up exercises (step 1). Then, choose from among the special-purpose qigong movements for brain and memory function, emotional balance, and nervous system and autonomic function (step 2). You need not do all of these movements to gain benefits. You can choose among them or do them all as time allows. At the beginning of your practice, it is sufficient to do just the warm-up and qigong exercises. But at some point, it is important to begin practicing taiji (step 3). Because taiji is not essential in the beginning of your practice, and because I have already covered taiji thoroughly in my book *Tai Chi in 10 Weeks: A Beginner's Guide* (YMAA, 2017), I will not present specific taiji exercises here. When you attain facility with the warm-up and qigong exercises, refer to that book and its companion video or find a good instructor in your area. As you begin practicing taiji, you may wish to reduce the number of warm-up and qigong exercises you do if you have time constraints. Finally, I offer a series of cool-down movements (step 4) to avoid the problems associated with the muscles going from warm to cool too quickly (we covered this in chapter 5).

After you practice, check yourself again for tension, weakness, and energy level. Do you still have fear or worries? What is your relaxation level now? Have these improved? Becoming conscious of these states will encourage and empower you to master your health and your life. You will become anchored in a new level of awareness and harmonize your brain multidimensionally, especially activating the frontal lobe.

Again, you do not have to do all of the movements described in this book. Feel free to choose only some of them, but certainly no harm will be done if you do them all.

Step 1: Total-Body Warm-Up Exercises

I discussed earlier that warm-up exercise is very important. I highly recommend doing the warm-up exercises below. They are designed for multiple health benefits and healing. But as we discussed earlier, you can also choose other warm-up exercises if you wish, such as power walking or jogging. Choose what works best for you.

I designed the following series of warm-up exercises to help your qi and blood flow through your whole body, loosen your muscles and joints, help your emotions, enhance your brain-cell communication, activate cross-activity between left brain and right brain, and promote organ harmony. This sequence of warm-up exercises involves whole-body movements. As I said before, you can go through all the movements or just some of them depending on how much time you have, your physical ability, or other circumstances. If you have trouble with certain movements, you can start out gently in the beginning and then gradually increase the intensity.

The warm-up can be done in fifteen to twenty minutes. If you have more problems in one area than others, you can focus on that area and devote more time to it.

Total-Body Twenty-Seven-Movement Warm-Up Exercises

The total-body twenty-seven-movement workout described below is designed for energy, blood circulation, balanced emotion, and brain stimulation. It should be practiced before taiji or qigong exercise.

1. ROCK FEET FORWARD AND BACKWARD

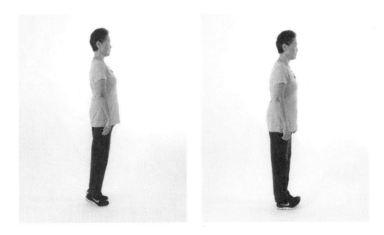

- Stand with your feet shoulder width apart and so your whole body is relaxed. Gently shift your weight to the balls of your feet, then from balls to the heels sixteen times without lift your feet off the ground.

2. ROCK FEET FORWARD AND BACKWARD, LIFTING HEELS

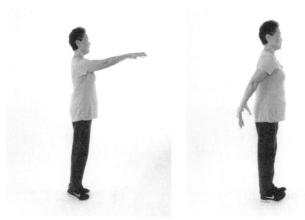

- Shift your weight to the balls of the feet and then to the heels as you did in exercise 1, but lift the heels and toes off the ground. As you shift back and forth, your arms and hands follow your body moving forward and backward. Do this sixteen times.

3. ALTERNATE SWINGING ARMS FORWARD AND BACKWARD

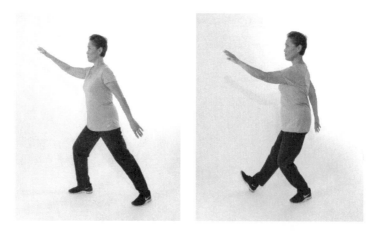

- Place your right leg in front of your left leg. Swing your arms forward and backward alternately as you shift weight from the front leg to the back leg. Your legs can be either straight or bent. Move one arm or both arms as you wish. Do eight swings on each side.

4. ROTATE SHOULDERS WHILE SHIFTING WEIGHT

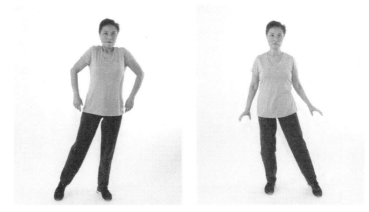

- Rotate the shoulders backward four times, then forward four times. As you rotate your shoulders, your chest moves too, and you shift your weight from one leg to the other. If you don't want to shift your weight, you can just rotate the shoulders. But when you rotate your shoulders while shifting weight, you get multidimension movements.

5. CIRCLE ARMS BACK AND FORTH (WHILE SHIFTING WEIGHT)

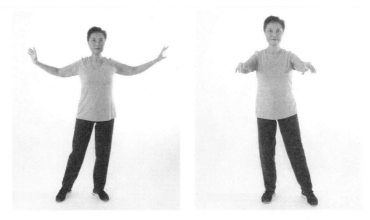

- Stand with your feet shoulder width apart. Make sure there is nothing within arm's length on any side of you. Extend your arms to the sides, and circle your arms backward eight times and forward eight times at moderate to fast speeds. As you circle, shift your weight from side to side. Make big circles like you are swimming. If you prefer, you can circle one arm at a time.

6. "WAX ON, WAX OFF" (VERTICAL, HORIZONTAL ARMS)

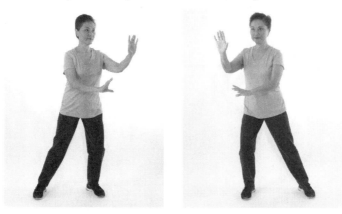

- With your palms facing forward, in a flexed position, alternately circle your arms in front of the body, like you are wiping off dirt from a wall. As you shift your weight to the left, your left hand circles outward from the middle of your chest to the left. Your right hand is in front of your abdomen. As you shift your weight to the right, your right hand circles outward from the middle of the chest to the right. Your left hand is in front of your abdomen. Do eight repetitions of this one too.

7. SIMPLE ARM PRESSING

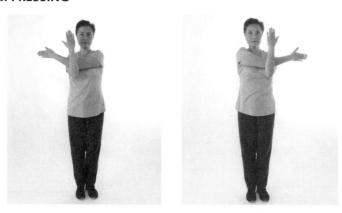

- Use your right forearm to press on your left upper arm in front of the body for three breaths. Then use your left forearm to press on your right upper arm in front of the body for three breaths.

8. PRESSING ARMS, MOVE UPPER BODY

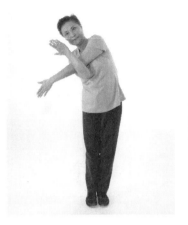
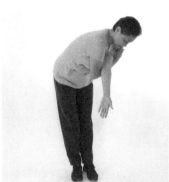

- Use your right forearm to press on your left upper arm in front of the body. Then move the body in a circle four times. Circle in the reverse direction four times. Next, use your left forearm to press on your right upper arm in front of the body, and circle in each direction four times.

9. WRIST ROTATION

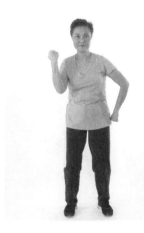
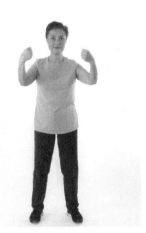

- Rotate your wrist one after the other, sixteen times for each wrist. You can move your body at the same time if you so desire. Do it freestyle with footwork—like dancing!

10. TENDON STRETCHING

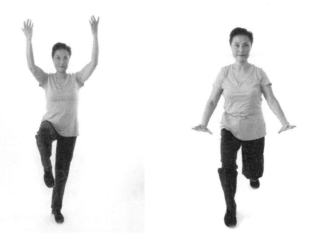

- Lift your hands and right leg. Then move the hands downward and put the right foot down in front of the body. The left foot is down with a slight lift of the heel. Stretch the left Achilles' tendon.

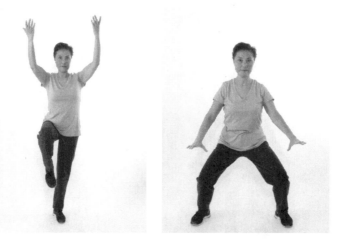

- Lift your hands and your right leg again, then place your right foot down next to left foot in a wide stance, and bend both legs, your arms lowering to hip level.

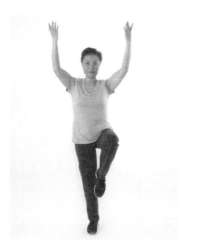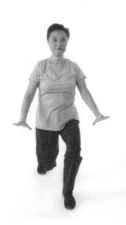

■ Lift your hands and left leg. Then move the hands downward, and put the left foot down in front of the body. The right foot is down with a slight lift of the heel. Stretch the right Achilles' tendon.

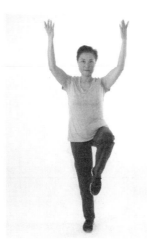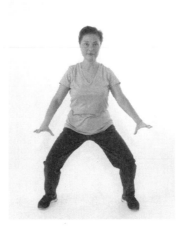

■ Lift your hands and your left leg again, then place your left foot down next to your right foot in a wide stance, and bend both legs, your arms lowering to hip level.

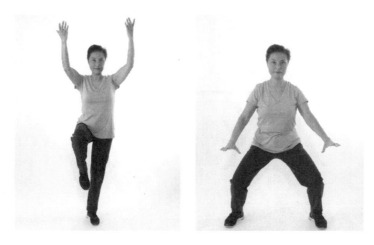

- Lift your hands and your right leg, then move your hands downward, and place your right foot to the side away from the left foot while you are stretching both Achilles' tendons.

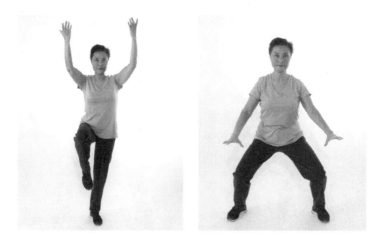

- Lift your hands and right leg again, and then place the right foot down next to the left foot, and bend both legs.

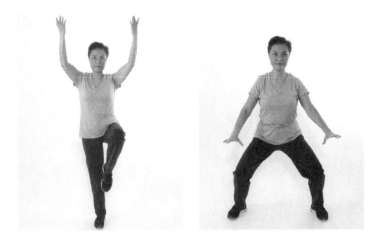

- Do the same with the left leg. Do this movement sequence eight times.

11. X-LIFTING

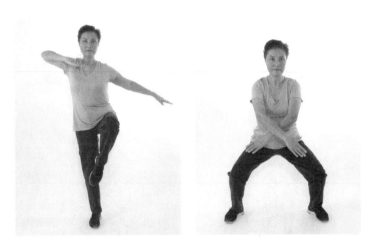

- Lift your right elbow and left foot. Put your left foot down as both forearms cross in front of the lower abdomen.

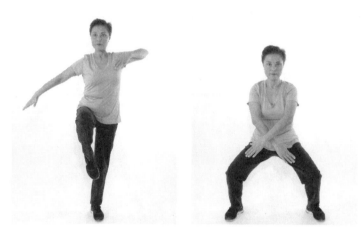

- Lift your left elbow and right foot. Put your right foot down as both forearms cross in front of the lower abdomen.
  Repeat eight times.

12. REACH SKY; TOUCH EARTH

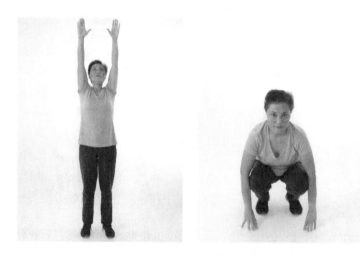

- With your feet either together or shoulder width apart, reach high with both hands, while rising onto your tiptoes if possible. Lower your heels until your feet are flat on the ground. Then with feet flat on the ground, bend your knees. Bend your body slowly over, and place both hands on the floor. It is not necessary to touch the floor if you are unable. Do eight repetitions.

13. Y ROTATION (FUNNEL CIRCLE)

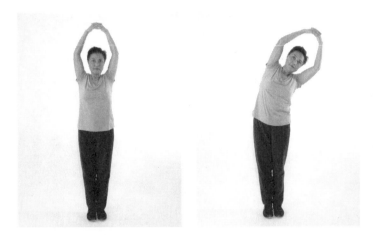

- Stand with your feet together, and stand straight with proper posture. Put your hands together above your head, with an imaginary string attached to them pulling upward so you feel that your body is lifted. Circle your hands while you keep your body still, like making an imaginary funnel over your head. Do four circles in each direction.

14. HIP ROTATION

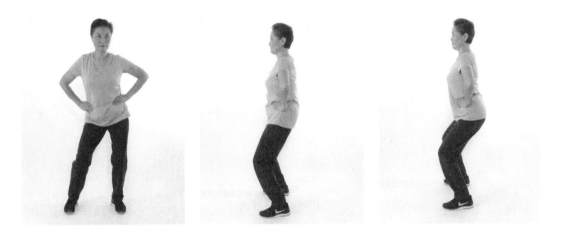

- Bend both legs slightly. Rotate hips clockwise four times, then counterclockwise four times. It's just like using a hula hoop but not as fast.

15. TOUCH OPPOSITE LEG AND FOOT

- Touch the opposite leg alternately. You might have done this movement in an aerobics class. The right hand touches the raised left leg, and then the left hand touches raised right leg. Do eight repetitions.

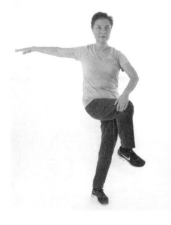

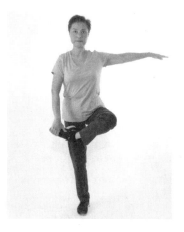

- Next, touch the opposite foot alternately. Right hand touches raised left foot. Left hand touches raised right foot. Do eight repetitions.

16. X-WALK FORWARD AND BACKWARD

This is really a nice movement you can do with music that has a moderate tempo. The rhythm and walk will make you feel uplifted and energized.

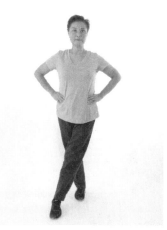

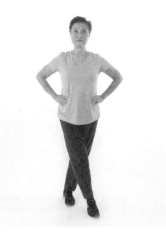

- Walk forward with the left foot crossing the right foot, then forward again with the right foot crossing the left foot four times. Do four of these forward left-right pairs. Then walk backward with the left foot crossing behind the right foot and then the right foot crossing behind the left foot. As with the forward movement, do this four times (just be careful of what's behind you!). Then repeat the whole sequence once more.

17. X-JUMP FORWARD AND BACKWARD

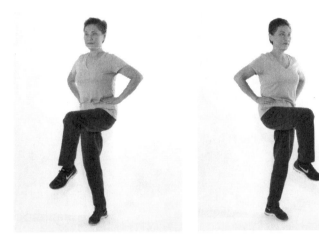

- In this exercise you jump instead of walk. Raise your left leg, and hop with your right. Then place your left foot down in front of your right. Raise your right leg, and hop on your left. Place right foot down in front of your left. Do this four times on each leg forward, then four times backward. This requires some coordination and no obstacles underfoot. Take precautions!

18. JUMP, CROSSING HANDS AND FEET

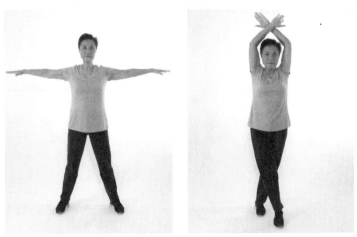

- Jump up once, and land with your feet a little more than shoulder width apart and arms straight out to your sides at shoulder level (open position). Jump again, crossing your right foot in front of your left foot while crossing your hands above your head.

- Next jump and land with the feet wide apart again, arms open at shoulder level. Jump again, crossing your left foot in front of your right foot, while you cross your hands in front of your lower abdomen. Repeat on the other side.
Repeat the sequence five to ten times or more.

19. JUMP, CROSSING HANDS HIGH AND FEET OPPOSITE

This movement is similar to the above, except now hands and feet cross at opposite times. This is kind of fun as it takes time to get the hang of it.

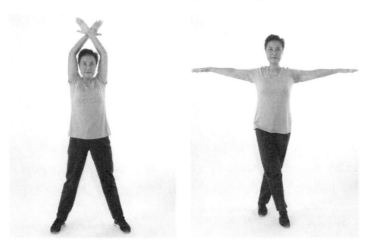

- This movement is just the opposite of the last one. Jump and land with your feet apart while crossing your arms over your head. Jump again and cross your right foot in front of your left foot, and open your arms to the side at shoulder level.
Jump again and land with your feet wide apart. This time, cross your hands over the lower abdomen. Jump again and cross your left foot in front of right, and open your arms to the sides at shoulder level. Repeat above five to ten more times.

20. KNOCKING METHOD MASSAGE

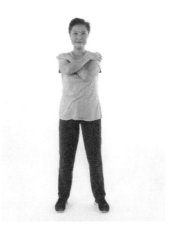

- Cross your hands.

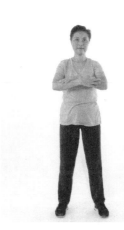 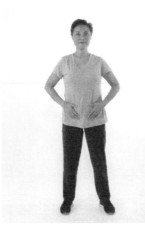 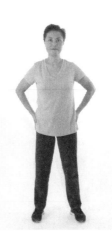

- Knock gently, with your arms crossed, on your shoulders, upper arms, forearms, and wrists. Then uncross your arms and gently knock on your head, hips, lower back, and legs. You should feel like you are waking up your whole body, part by part.

21. AIRPLANE

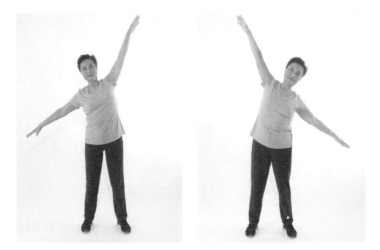

- It sounds a little exotic, but it is easy to do. Place your arms out to your sides at shoulder level. Move the body in a circle while keeping the arms still. Do four circles to each side.

22. BUDDHA HOLDING QI

- Stand in horse stance, with your feet wide apart, knees bent, and pelvis tucked under. Position your arms to the side of the body, below shoulder level, with the palms up. Relax your whole body. Focus on deep and slow breathing. You can have your eyes closed or open. Focus your mind on your hands, and relax your lower back. Hold for three breaths or more if you are able.

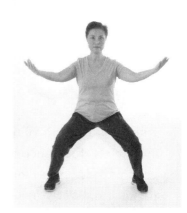

23. SIDE LUNGE, ALTERNATELY SHIFTING WEIGHT

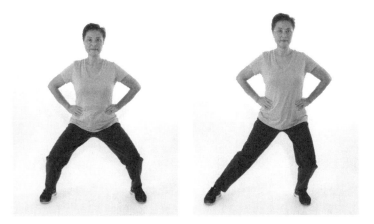

- Start in horse stance (see last movement). Slowly shift your weight to your left, and hold for three breaths, then to your right, holding for three breaths.

24. UPSIDE-DOWN Y WITH DEEP BREATHING

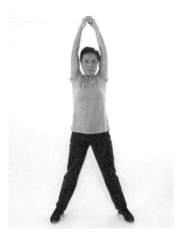

- Stand with your feet apart, two times your shoulder width, with legs straight. Interlock your fingers above your head with the arms straight. Focus on deep breathing.

25. LUNGE AND BEND FORWARD

- Step into a forward
  lunge with your right
  foot. Take a deep
  breath, and raise
  your hands above
  your head. Exhale
  and move your hands
  down to the floor,
  keeping both legs
  straight if you can.
  Repeat four times.

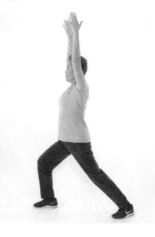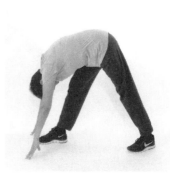

Lunge forward with your left foot. Inhale and raise your hands above your head. Exhale and move your hands down to the floor, keeping both legs straight if you can. Repeat four times.

26. CHINESE "BIG," DEEP BREATHING

If you know the Chinese character for *big* [大], you'll have no problem doing this movement.

- Stand with your feet
  apart, two times your
  shoulder width. Place
  your arms out to
  your sides at
  shoulder level, and
  breathe through the
  body. With your
  palms facing down,
  focus your mind on

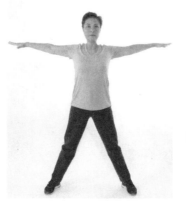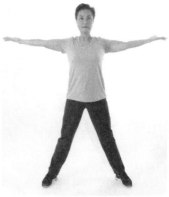

your palms, and imagine them drawing energy from the earth. Inhale and exhale this energy ten times. Turn your palms to face up. Focus your mind on your palms, and imagine them filling with energy from the sun and the universe. Inhale and exhale this energy ten times.

27. SHAKE HANDS AND FEET, ENDING

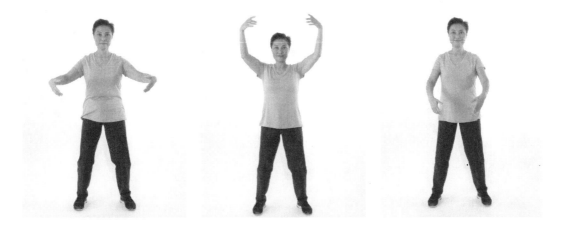

- Shake your hands vigorously for ten to twenty seconds. Next, shake your arms and body vigorously.

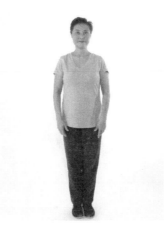

- Take three deep breaths, and bow to yourself and the world in thanks. You have finished the total-body warm-up practice!

Step 2: Qigong Practice for Special Purposes

Qigong Exercises for Brain and Memory

This exercise group helps to balance both sides of the brain, the upper and lower parts of the brain, as well as the midbrain. These exercises, when performed in conjunction with taiji practice, enhance brain efficiency and memory. When I do these exercises regularly, I can really feel the difference in my mental processes, emotions, and memory. The results are often immediate.

1. MOVE QI THROUGH YOUR BODY

■ Stand with your feet shoulder width apart. Raise your arms up the sides of the body, and then bring the arms down in front of the body. As you are doing this movement, imagine that you are gathering universal energy and allowing it to go through your body. Repeat three to five times.

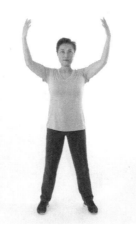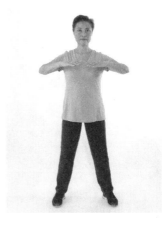

2. PUSH UP; OPEN THE SKY

■ Inhale and raise your arms up in front of the body as if you are pushing up a weight. Visualize lifting the energy from the earth and letting it move through your body, through your head, and connecting that energy with the heavens.

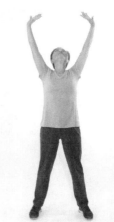

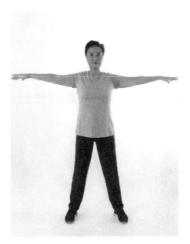

- Exhale and open and lower your arms to the sides. While lowering your arms, open yourself to the energy of the universe. Bring the arms all the way down, next to your legs. Repeat five times.

3. SHIFT BODY WEIGHT SIDE TO SIDE, REACHING

This practice helps to balance yin and yang. It also creates the effective communication between the left and right hemispheres of the brain (including the frontal lobe and the sensory motor cortexes), as well as the left and right sides of the body.

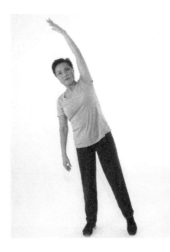 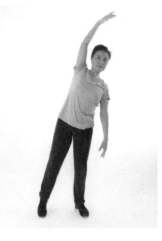

- Stand with your body in a proper posture with the feet shoulder width apart. Shift your weight to the right and reach your left arm up over your head to the right. Next, perform this movement to the opposite side. Do eight to each side for a total of sixteen.

4. HORIZONTAL 8, MOVING THE BALL

This is a taiji skill practice for left and right brain hemispheres.

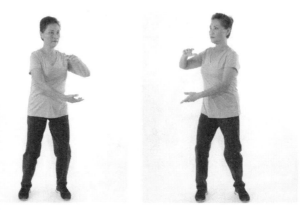

- Put one hand above the other, like you are holding a basketball. Turn your body toward the side of your upper hand. Then exchange the position of your hands while turning your body to the opposite side. It looks like you are moving the ball in a horizontal figure eight. Do eight on each side for a total of sixteen.

5. TOUCH SKY; TOUCH EARTH

This movement is checking your center dimensionality, as well as working to stimulate the midbrain. It helps to move qi through the body more efficiently. When you touch the floor, you stretch your Achilles' tendon while your natural posture performs massage on your internal organs.

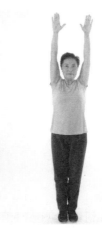

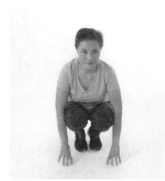

- Inhale as you reach high with both hands. Then bend your knees, and touch the floor as you exhale. You can do eight repetitions or up to twenty.

6. ROCK FEET, FRONT AND BACK

We mentioned this movement previously. This is a good balance practice. This gentle movement is checking focus dimension, working with the brain stem and cerebellum. You can either just rock back and forth or rise onto your toes and heels while you are rocking.

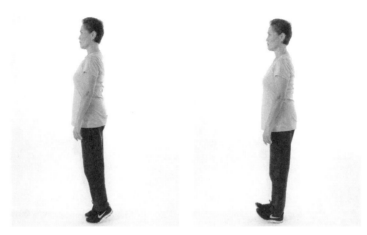

- Shift your weight to the balls of the feet and then to the heels as you did in exercise 1, but lift the heels and toes higher. As you shift back and forth, your arms and hands follow your body moving forward and backward. Do sixteen repetitions.

7. X-POSE

X-pose is an excellent qi practice, as well as a brain exercise. It allows all your channels to open so your body can receive energy from the universe through them.

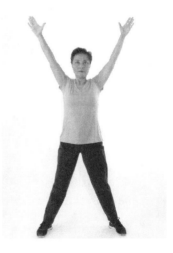

- Stand with your feet apart two times your shoulder width. Raise your arms above your head and open wide so your whole body makes the letter X. Inhale and exhale deeply five times.

8. FOLDING X-POSE

- Stand in the standing X-pose. Bend your body forward, and put your hands on your feet. Hold for three breaths.

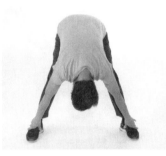

9. TWO-DIMENSION X-POSE

This is also an excellent brain exercise, working on space orientation.

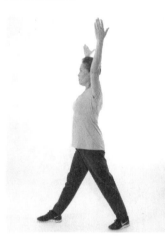

- Stand with one foot in front. Raise your arms above your head and open wide, so your whole body makes the letter *X*. Inhale and exhale deeply five times, then repeat on the other side.

10. FOLDING TWO-DIMENSION X-POSE

This is also an excellent brain workout for improved space orientation.

- While you're in the two-dimension twisted X-pose, slowly bend forward until you touch the floor. If you have to bend your front knee when you touch the floor, that's OK. Hold for three breaths, then repeat on the other side.

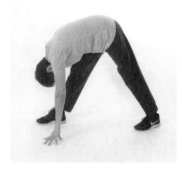

11. CIRCLE KNEES IN TWO DIRECTIONS

This coordinated legwork takes a lot of practice to master. If you practice often, you can do it. This is not only an excellent brain workout because it involves multiple brain tasks, but it is also an excellent joint exercise. Don't you love things with multiple benefits?

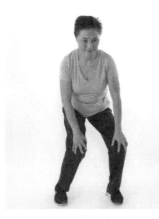 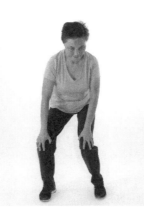

- Simultaneously circle your knees in opposite directions. The movement of each leg is not mirroring the other but rather, following in a similar but opposite motion. Circle eight times in each direction.

12. HEAD MASSAGE

There are many meridians and points that go through the head; these meridians are related to the brain and brain chemicals. By stimulating them with massage, you send signals to the brain and brain cells, increasing brain communication.

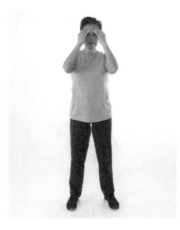 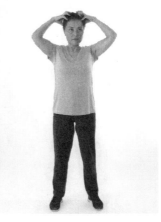

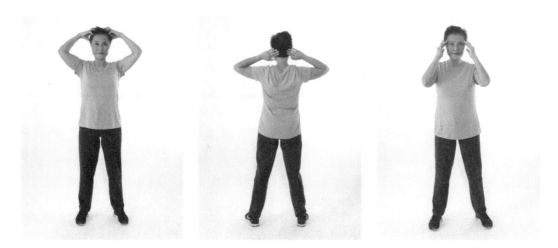

- Massage your forehead and temple area; the top, back, and base of the scalp; and then your whole head. Massage for one to two minutes.

13. NECK MOVEMENT

The neck is one of the most important structures in the body. There are many important structures that go through the neck. The blood vessels go to your brain; the nervous system goes to your brain; the nervous system goes to your arms and upper body, the lymphatic system, the cervical discs, and the central nervous system; and all have a relationship (connection) with your neck. Cervical health is very important to your overall health.

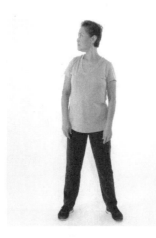
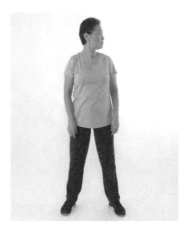

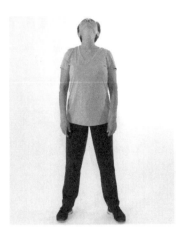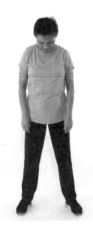

- Slowly turn your head to the left, to the right, up, and down. Your eyes always follow in the direction of each movement. Repeat eight times.

14. IN-MOTION HOOKUP

This movement has multiple benefits: brain exercise, qi exercise, coordination exercise, stretching, and more. This movement is not easy to do in the beginning; but once you get it, it is very easy to do.

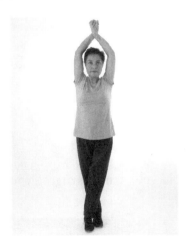

- Cross your feet and hands. Rotate your wrists so they face each other with the hands crossed, and interlock the fingers. Inhale, and raise your hands over your head.

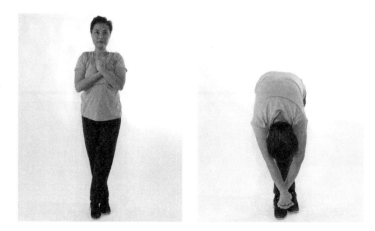

- Inhale and raise your body as you rotate your hands inward until they are at the front of your chest. Then exhale, bending forward as you point your hands downward toward the floor.

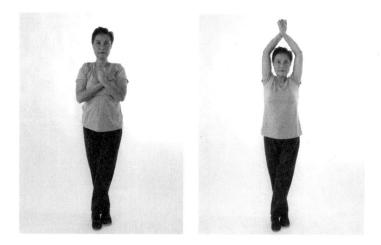

- Inhale. Raise your body and your arms, bringing your arms overhead. Hold this position for a breath or two.

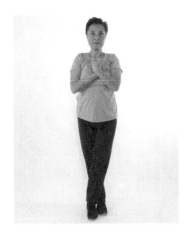

- Exhale as you lower your arms to the front of your body with your fingers interlocked. Inhale rotate your interlocked hands and as you rotate your hands inward, and then exhale, bending forward as you point them downward toward the floor.

- Drop your hands, uncross your feet, and relax your shoulders and your whole body. Repeat this motion four times.

Qigong Exercises for Emotional Balance

There are many people who suffer with emotional issues stemming from various causes. There is not much a doctor can do besides prescribe medication. Our culture does not do much to help either, but you can help yourself by performing some specific exercises and doing them regularly. Or you can do them as needed. Emotional issues are related to a brain chemical imbalance. In Chinese medicine theory, these issues stem from organ disharmony—or, as I like to say, from "lost organ teamwork." The movements stimulate the meridian system, circulation system, and the brain, all of which help to balance your brain chemicals. You feel better every time you do these exercises. If you don't feel like doing these exercises, you can just walk outside, swinging your arms widely. This will also bring great benefits. The worst thing you can do to yourself is to be a couch potato, which will make you feel stuck. If you move your body, you may be surprised at how your emotions change. There are also very good Chinese herbal medicines that can help with emotional problems.

This group of qigong movements helps to relieve anxiety, depression, high stress caused by emotional imbalance, and panic attacks. Some of these movements have been explained previously.

1. TURN BODY FROM SIDE TO SIDE

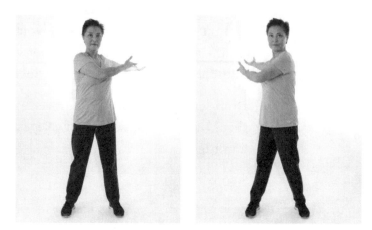

- Stand with your feet shoulder width apart. Stand straight with arms and neck relaxed. Turn your upper body from side to side, allowing your arms to swing freely. Repeat this as many times as you like.

2. RELEASE LIVER ENERGY

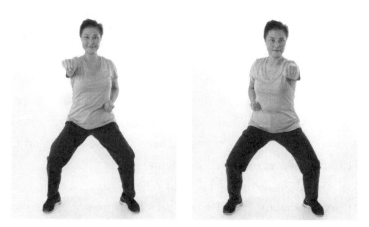

- Stand in the horse stance position—feet wide apart, knees bent, and pelvis tucked under. Inhale and put both fists at waist level. Exhale and quickly, but without jerking your shoulders, move your right fist forward, like you are punching a ball in front of you. Inhale and bring your right fist back to your waist. Exhale and quickly move your left fist forward. Repeat this as many times as you want.

3. STANDING X-POSE (OPEN ALL CHANNELS)

As we discussed before, X-pose is an excellent qi practice as well as brain exercise. Because this pose allows all channels to open, your body receives energy from the universe through the channels as you focus on deep breathing. Opening your energy channels helps to remove the stagnation that causes emotional problems.

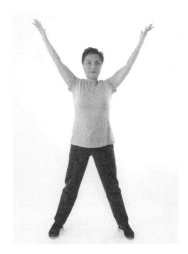

- Stand with your feet apart two times your shoulder width. Raise your arms above your head and open wide, so your whole body makes the letter *X*. Inhale and exhale deeply five times.

4. CHINESE "BIG," PALMS UP

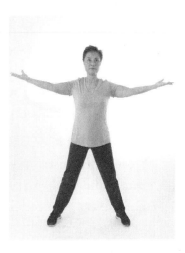

- Stand with your feet apart, two times your shoulder width. Place your arms out to your sides at shoulder level, and breathe through the body. With your palms facing up, imagine them filling with energy from the sun and the universe. Breathe slowly and deeply. Each time you inhale, the energy goes smoothly to your palms; each time you exhale, the energy goes through your body to your arms, chest, lower abdomen, legs, and feet. Then the energy returns to the earth from your feet. You may close your eyes while performing this movement. Do this movement for two to five minutes as you wish, or anytime you need to.

5. CHINESE "BIG," PALMS DOWN

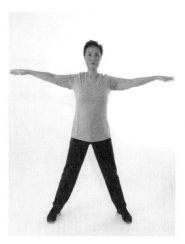

- With your palms facing down, focus your mind on your palms, and imagine them drawing energy from the earth. As you inhale, draw energy from the earth to your palms. As you exhale, imagine the energy going through your body. Then connect to earth energy through your feet.

6. CONNECT UPPER AND LOWER DAN TIAN

There are several dan tian points in the body, all very important focal points for your center of gravity and your overall energy health. This position concerns the dan tian points at your heart center and below your navel.

- Put your right hand on your sternum (in the center of your chest just above your solar plexus) and your left hand on your lower abdomen. Focus your mind on the connection between these two energy centers while breathing in and breathing slowly five to ten times.

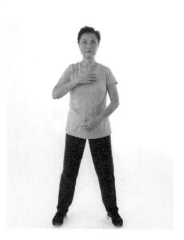

7. CROSS HANDS AND FEET

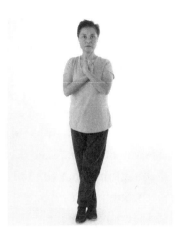

- Cross your wrists and interlock your fingers. Put one foot across the front of the other. Take a deep breath as you turn your wrists inward. Breathe out, and continue to rotate your wrists until your elbows point downward and your hands point upward. Relax your shoulders, elbows, and wrists. Keep your fingers interlocked, and hold for five breaths; then switch hands and feet, and hold for five more breaths.

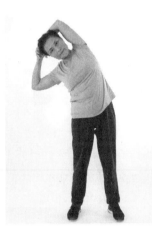

8. GRAB HAND BEHIND HEAD; BEND SIDEWAYS

- Take a deep breath, and use your right hand to grab your left wrist behind your head. Breathe out, and lean your body to the right. After two breaths, relax your body and arms, and return to standing straight.

- Take a deep breath, and use your left hand to grab your right wrist behind your head. Breathe out, and lean your body to the left. After two breaths, relax your body and arms, and return to standing straight. Repeat two or three times on both sides.

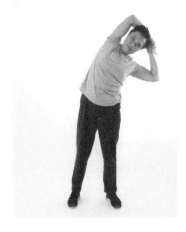

9. Y BLOSSOM

This requires your mind to be present and to focus on your body and breath.

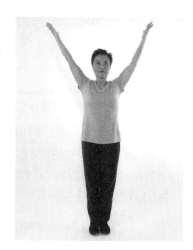

- Stand with your feet together and your arms up and open in a Y shape. Your feet are rooted and receive energy from the earth. Your arms are straight and relaxed. Breathe deeply and slowly, imagining that you are receiving universal energy through your fingers and hands, that it goes through your arms and body and connects with earth energy. Hold for at least three breaths.

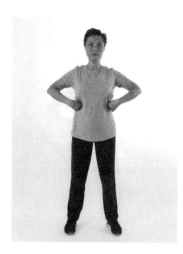

10. ACUPRESSURE LIVER POINT

- Put your hands at the side of your chest with thumbs on the front of your rib cage and fingers at the back. With the tips of your thumbs and support from your forefingers, find the point that feels sensitive, and press on it. Then massage gently by circling your arms.

11. ARM MASSAGE

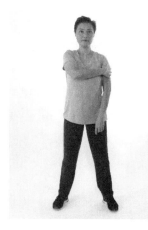

- There are six meridians that go through the arms, three meridians on each side, with many energy points. These meridians connect to your organs. When you massage the arms, you are actually stimulating these meridians and points. Use one hand to massage the whole length of the opposite arm. Change hands and arms after about three minutes.

12. EAR MASSAGE

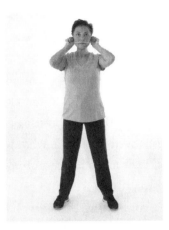

- Your ears are like a miniature body. They have many points that correspond to various body parts. Massage your ears, and you are indirectly massaging your whole body. Do this for about three minutes.

13. SIDE BODY BEND

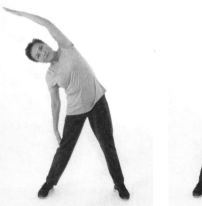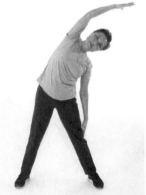

- Stand with your feet apart, arms straight out to the sides. Bend your body to the right with the left arm extended over your head to the right. Hold this position for three breaths. Then bend your body to the left with the right arm extended over your head to the left. Hold for three breaths.

Qigong Exercises for Nervous System and Autonomic Function

The nervous system is a very complicated system that can cause many health issues if not appropriately cared for. To keep the nervous system healthy, just keeping a healthy mind is not enough. For example, some people are very spiritual and positive, which is a good thing, but if they have a sedentary lifestyle and do not exercise, sooner or later they will have health issues. The components of the body must be kept alive, active, and moving because they influence our nervous system. This is what we call mind and body wellness. Keeping our nervous system healthy is a key to preventing illness.

By looking at the following pictures, we can see how the nervous system affects everything in the body. The key to keeping the nervous system healthy is to keep the spine healthy. For this reason, appropriate exercise for the spine is crucial for maintaining a healthy nervous system.

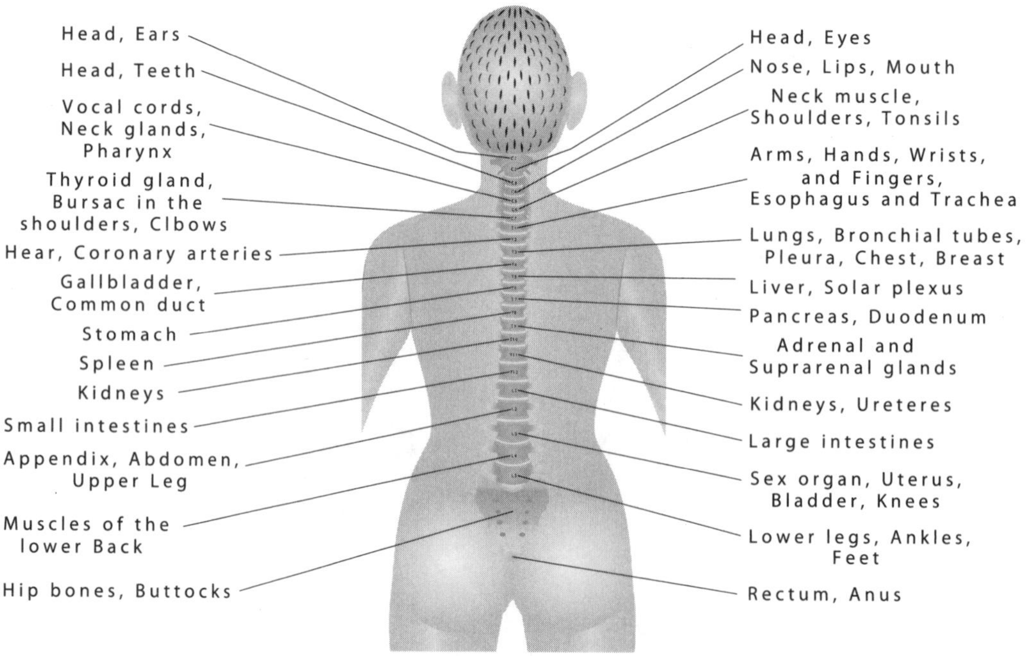

Head, Ears
Head, Teeth
Vocal cords, Neck glands, Pharynx
Thyroid gland, Bursac in the shoulders, Clbows
Hear, Coronary arteries
Gallbladder, Common duct
Stomach
Spleen
Kidneys
Small intestines
Appendix, Abdomen, Upper Leg
Muscles of the lower Back
Hip bones, Buttocks
Head, Eyes
Nose, Lips, Mouth
Neck muscle, Shoulders, Tonsils
Arms, Hands, Wrists, and Fingers, Esophagus and Trachea
Lungs, Bronchial tubes, Pleura, Chest, Breast
Liver, Solar plexus
Pancreas, Duodenum
Adrenal and Suprarenal glands
Kidneys, Ureteres
Large intestines
Sex organ, Uterus, Bladder, Knees
Lower legs, Ankles, Feet
Rectum, Anus

Nervous System
Image by Iotan/Shutterstock

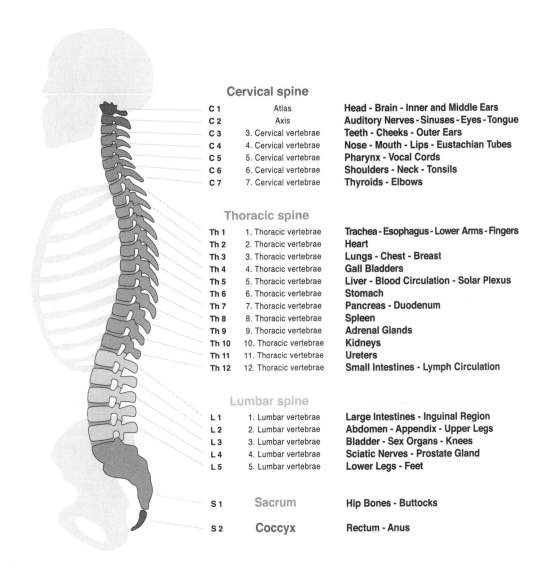

Cervical spine

C 1	Atlas	Head - Brain - Inner and Middle Ears
C 2	Axis	Auditory Nerves - Sinuses - Eyes - Tongue
C 3	3. Cervical vertebrae	Teeth - Cheeks - Outer Ears
C 4	4. Cervical vertebrae	Nose - Mouth - Lips - Eustachian Tubes
C 5	5. Cervical vertebrae	Pharynx - Vocal Cords
C 6	6. Cervical vertebrae	Shoulders - Neck - Tonsils
C 7	7. Cervical vertebrae	Thyroids - Elbows

Thoracic spine

Th 1	1. Thoracic vertebrae	Trachea - Esophagus - Lower Arms - Fingers
Th 2	2. Thoracic vertebrae	Heart
Th 3	3. Thoracic vertebrae	Lungs - Chest - Breast
Th 4	4. Thoracic vertebrae	Gall Bladders
Th 5	5. Thoracic vertebrae	Liver - Blood Circulation - Solar Plexus
Th 6	6. Thoracic vertebrae	Stomach
Th 7	7. Thoracic vertebrae	Pancreas - Duodenum
Th 8	8. Thoracic vertebrae	Spleen
Th 9	9. Thoracic vertebrae	Adrenal Glands
Th 10	10. Thoracic vertebrae	Kidneys
Th 11	11. Thoracic vertebrae	Ureters
Th 12	12. Thoracic vertebrae	Small Intestines - Lymph Circulation

Lumbar spine

L 1	1. Lumbar vertebrae	Large Intestines - Inguinal Region
L 2	2. Lumbar vertebrae	Abdomen - Appendix - Upper Legs
L 3	3. Lumbar vertebrae	Bladder - Sex Organs - Knees
L 4	4. Lumbar vertebrae	Sciatic Nerves - Prostate Gland
L 5	5. Lumbar vertebrae	Lower Legs - Feet
S 1	Sacrum	Hip Bones - Buttocks
S 2	Coccyx	Rectum - Anus

Spine and Level of Correlated Spinal Nerve
Image by Peter Hermes Furian/Shutterstock

As you see, the nervous system is related to all parts of our body. The nervous system has also been at the center of my lifetime of practice. I focus on tuning it up and keeping it functioning smoothly. The traditional Chinese medicine meridian system has a very close relationship with the nervous system.

1. TURN BODY AND SWING ARMS FROM SIDE TO SIDE

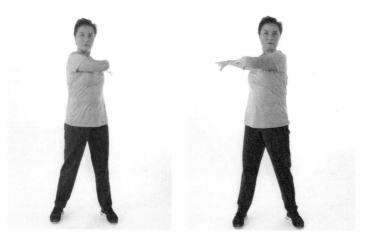

- Stand with your feet shoulder width apart. Keep your weight in the center while turning your body from side to side, swinging your arms with the movement. Keep your head relaxed and straight (do not turn your head while turning your body). Turn eight times in each direction.

2. BIG SHOULDER ROLL

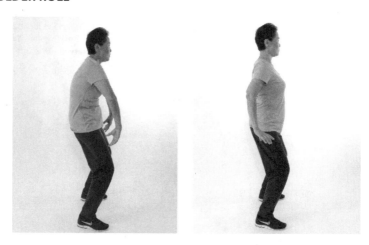

- Take a deep breath. When you breathe out, roll your shoulders forward. Inhale and roll your shoulders upward. Exhale and roll your shoulders backward. Now inhale and roll your shoulders upward, and exhale, rolling your shoulders forward and down. Repeat this eight times.

3. BIG SHOULDER ROTATION

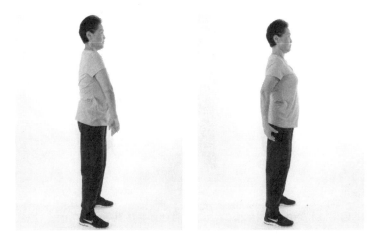

- Rotate your shoulders forward four times, then backward four times. Inhale when you rotate shoulders upward, and exhale when you rotate shoulders downward.

4. NECK MOVEMENT AND ROTATION

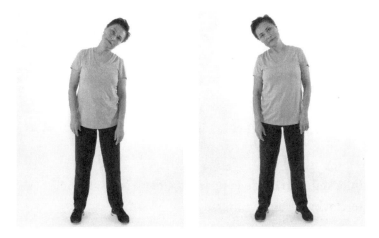

- Slowly lower your left ear toward your left shoulder, then slowly lower your right ear toward your right shoulder. Repeat eight times.

    Tilt your head down, and roll your head from left to right and then from right to left. Do this eight times.

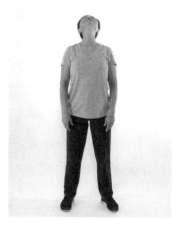

- Tilt your head back, and roll your head from left to right and then from right to left. Do this eight times.

5. HIP ROTATION

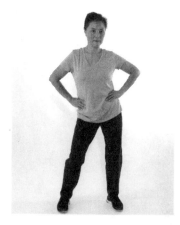 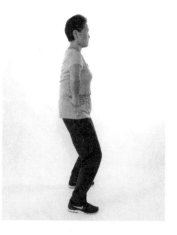 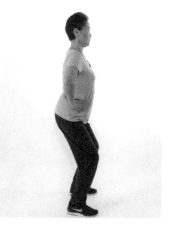

- Keep legs unlocked, and circle your waist clockwise eight times. Then circle your waist counterclockwise eight times.

6. VERTICAL HIP ROTATION

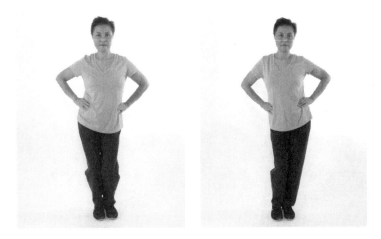

- Place your feet together. Circle your hip up and down from right to left four times, then left to right four times.

7. DANCING (STATIONARY OR WALKING)

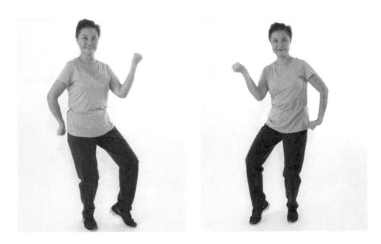

- Dance with your hips moving with a fun attitude. Free your spirit, and free your body. You feel good when you move with a free mind and body. Dance for at least one minute.

8. SWIMMING PRACTICE (ARCH BACK FORWARD AND BACKWARD)

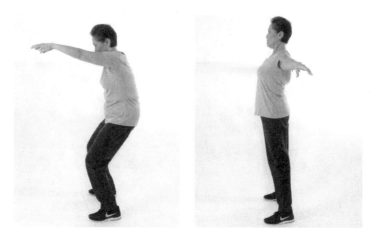

- Place your arms to the side of your body. Inhale, circling your arms inward toward the body. Arch your back as you exhale, circling your arms out to the side in a continuous motion. Inhale. Do this sequence eight times.

9. REACH TO THE SIDE (KEEP HIPS STILL)

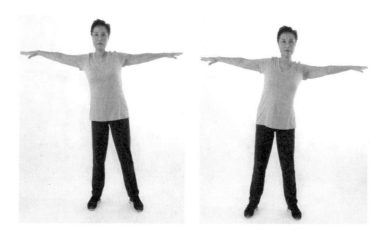

- Keep your hips still and your arms straight out to your sides. Alternately shift the upper body right and left, while you keep your hips in the center. Do eight repetitions on each side for a total of sixteen.

10. Y ROTATION (FUNNEL CIRCLE)

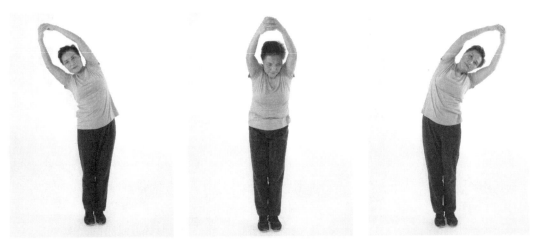

- We saw this exercise in the warm-up section and will repeat it here because it is an important movement for the spine and nervous system. Grab your hands over your head. Circle the upper body while you keep the legs straight. Repeat four times in each direction.

11. CIRCLE ARMS IN OPPOSITE DIRECTIONS

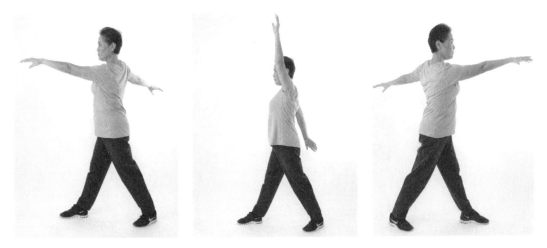

- Make a full circle with your left arm clockwise in front of your body, turning your body along with the movement, then in the back of your body on the left make a circle counterclockwise. Your right arm moves in the opposite direction of the left arm. Do four repetitions. Next, make a full circle counterclockwise with your right hand in front of your body, then toward the back on your right side, clockwise. Your left arm moves in the opposite direction of the right arm. Do four repetitions to the right as well.

The movement is like drawing a somewhat folded number eight. It also helps to visualize a clock on the wall in front of you.

12. BEND FORWARD AND RELAX, ENDING

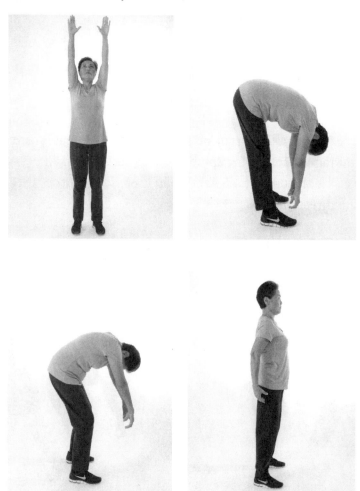

- Take a deep breath, and raise your hands over your head. Exhale as you bend forward, lowering your body fully, and relax the entire upper body. Hold for three breaths. Then roll up, and end standing up straight.

Step 3: Taiji Practice

Although we will not discuss specific taiji exercises in this book, I do wish to mention here that taiji is particularly good for brain health. It helps you to quiet your mind and regulate your breath. Regulating your breath not only allows your brain to rest but also brings more oxygen to the body and brain through deep breathing. In addition, the special movements of taiji stimulate and activate all parts of the brain. This is why people who practice taiji regularly show well-rounded living skills: balanced emotions, intuition, cognitive function, problem-solving skills, ability to learn quickly, logical decision-making, and organization.

Step 4: Cool-Down Movements

Whatever exercise you do, you should always do some stretching and other body movements to cool down afterward. You will be more relaxed, and your energy channels will be opened. An appropriate cooldown also helps to ensure that you get the most benefit possible from the exercise.

Ten-Step Cooldown

1. REACH UP

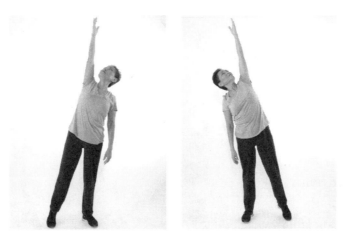

- Raise one hand as high as you can as you inhale. Your weight is on the opposite foot. Exhale as you relax and lower the arm and hand. As you inhale, raise your other hand as high as you can, and shift your weight onto the opposite foot. Exhale as you relax the body and drop the arm and hand. Do this four times.

2. STRETCH QUADRICEPS

- Lift your left foot behind your buttock. Use one or two hands to grab your foot and bring it close to your buttock. Stretch for three breaths, then change sides.

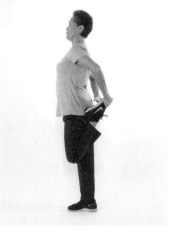

3. STRETCH HAMSTRINGS

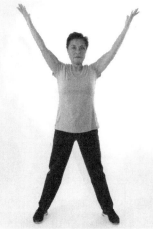

- Place your left foot in front of you with the heel down and toe up. Bend forward. Keep the left leg straight and the right leg bent, and try to grab your left toes (or just try to get as close as you can). Hold for three breaths, then repeat on the right side.

4. BEND FORWARD, HANDS TOUCHING THE FLOOR

- Take a deep breath, and raise your hands above your head. Breathe out as you bend forward. Put your hands on the floor if you can. Hold for three breaths.

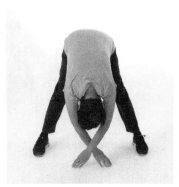

5. FRONT LUNGE, STRETCHING HIP

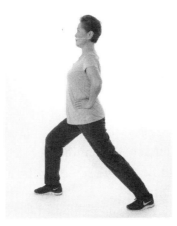

- Take a big step forward with your left foot. Shift your weight to the front leg, bending at the knee. Hold for three breaths, then change to the other foot and do the same thing.

6. FLOOR STRETCHING

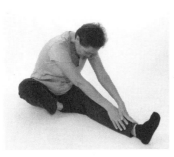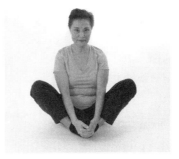

- Floor stretching can vary. You can use yoga postures if you are familiar with them. If you are unfamiliar with stretching techniques, you can use the ones pictured. In the first, place one foot against the inner thigh of the opposite leg, and slowly move your upper body toward your straight leg, holding your leg and stretching for at least three breaths. Repeat on the other side. Next, press your feet together and draw them as close to your body as possible. At the same time, try to press the knees to the ground. Hold for at least three breaths.

The best way to find what you need is to pay attention to which part of your body is tight or aches.

7. SELF-MASSAGE ON LEG

- In a sitting position, you can easily massage your legs with your elbow. Massage for about two minutes. Now do the same for the other leg.

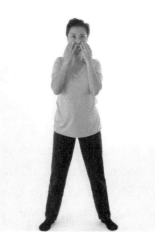

8. KNEE SITTING

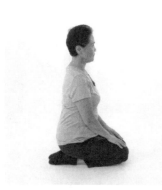

- This position is often seen in Japanese culture. It stretches the stomach meridian and also relaxes the lower back, allowing spinal fluid to flow more easily. Stay in this position for two to three minutes. While you are sitting, continue to practice deep breathing and focus on energy flowing through your spine.

9. SELF-MASSAGE OF FOREHEAD, FACE, AND NECK

- Continue in the knee sitting position (or stand as pictured) and massage your forehead and temple

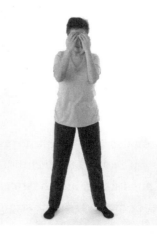

for a minute. Then massage your face for a minute. Next, massage your neck for a minute.

10. ENDING WITH DEEP BREATHING AND FULL RELAXATION

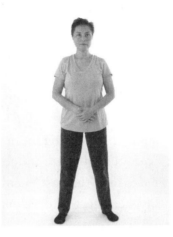

- Breathe slowly and deeply. Be aware that all parts of your body are relaxed. If you still feel some tension, continue to breathe until you feel the full sensation of relaxation. Do this for one to two minutes.

Final Words

If you are stressed, move your body.

If you feel imbalanced, move your body.

If you feel fog in your brain, move your body.

If you have ailments no one can help, move your body.

If you are forgetful, move your body.

If there is anything that is troubling you, move your body.

Chapter 7

Where Am I on My Path?

WE GET DISTRACTED easily by all kinds of things. As we are just about to make a positive change, something else gets in the way. We often make excuses for not doing what is in our own best interests, especially when it comes to our health. We all know what to do and how to do it. But we don't know how to be persistent. I too am often distracted by so many things going on in my life. Fortunately, because of my taiji and qigong habit, I can quickly catch up on things I am supposed to be doing. I have taught many students over the past twenty years, and those who have been diligent about their learning, healing, and development have made real changes in their lives.

Learning, healing, and developing the mind, body, and spirit takes time and effort. It requires dedication and determination. It is a lifestyle commitment, a total life revolution.

Remember also to always listen to your inner wisdom. It will teach you what is going on with you and how to make things better. I had a patient who was going through some hard times and was under tremendous stress. She was seeing many different doctors, holistic practitioners, and even acupuncturists for her health issues, but nothing seemed to work. She was upset, angry, confused, stressed, and tired of searching for answers in all different directions. For a long time, she faithfully followed every instruction given by her doctors, therapists, and acupuncturists. But eventually, she realized that all these medical professionals were saying different things, and this made her more confused. I finally had to ask her, "How much did you listen to *yourself*?"

She replied, "Not at all."

I asked her, "Do you know what is really going on with your health?"

She said, "No, that is why I am going to all these practitioners and doctors!"

She had lost all sense of what was going on in her own life and health. Her energy was totally chaotic, going in as many different directions as the number of healing methods she was trying. Her brain's network was tangled, and her brain cells were not communicating with each other in an efficient way. She could not breathe, suffocated by all this stress. Her confused mind could not make logical decisions about her healing path.

If this had been twenty years ago, I would have raised my voice and yelled, "Wake up, move, breathe, or get lost!" Instead, I gave her a big hug and told her to follow her instincts to find out what was causing her stress. I guided her to let go of the thoughts that were troubling her. I provided treatment to her with affection and in a way that was natural, nurturing, and caring. I couldn't help but notice that I too had improved over the years—I think I was a little snobby twenty years ago, don't you?

We should look at the course of our lives to see where our paths are leading. Whether you are a left-brainer or a right-brainer, you can always make a difference. The difference is that you are always smarter than others about one thing: yourself.

I made this self-checklist for your convenience, but you need not use it if you have already developed the discipline of self-awareness.

Self-Checklist

This is a self-assessment to find out where your practice has taken you. Rate your answers on a 1–5 scale, with the most positive being a 5 and the least positive a 1. Don't put expectations on your score; when you've practiced for a long time, you may get a 5. But if you get a low score, it is not necessarily a bad thing. It just means you need to practice more regularly and persistently. Nothing is impossible. Just open your mind to the possibilities. Think about doing this self-check once a month to know yourself better. Remember, as long as you put your mind to it, you will become what you are born to be and get everything you want.

1. Do I practice every day?

2. Am I focused when I am practicing these exercises?

3. Am I focused overall?

4. How is my balance overall?

5. How do I feel after each practice?

6. How was the tension in my body during practice?

7. How was the tension in my mind during practice?

8. How well have I been able to deal with stress?

9. How well have I been able to function in social environments?

10. Is my memory getting better?

11. How is my learning ability?

12. How is my reading? Is it faster than before?

13. Am I solving problems better?

14. How are my relationships with others?

15. Am I willing to explore more new things than before?

16. Am I able to do all the movements correctly?

17. How is my level of understanding of qi?

18. Do I feel the qi?

19. How is my confidence level?

20. What is my stress level?

21. What is my relaxation level?

22. How are my emotions when facing certain situations?

23. Am I calmer in general, better than before?

24. Am I more aware of my energy now, more than before?

25. Am I more willing to share my experience with others?

26. How is my mental creativity?

27. Do I have a goal now?

28. What is my goal now?

29. Am I generally stronger than before?

30. What is my fear level now? Is it less than before?

31. What is my ultimate goal, and will I reach it?

32. Do I agree with the following statements?

    o I am strong.

    o I can do anything I wish.

    o I can learn anything I wish.

    o I can heal myself.

    o I can change.

    o I am very confident about myself.

Conclusion

HAVING LIVED in United States for almost thirty years and having worked with many patients including children, I have noticed that there is an urgent need: *natural health education should start at an early age.* I have seen so many children using medications when they could instead be helped in a natural way. Children with weight problems, emotional problems, and other physical ailments can be helped with natural methods. Many adult problems come from childhood issues. Some had an unhealthy diet, and some were given too many medications, among other things.

Here are a few suggestions you should keep in mind:

- When your mind and emotions are stuck, move your body and do structured movement exercises.
- When you feel depressed or anxious, move your body and do structured movement exercises.
- When your healing is poor or just not happening, move your body and, if you are able, do structured movement exercises.
- When you cannot use your mind anymore, use your body.

Here are a few things to remember:

- If you focus on disease, you have disease.
- If you focus on problems, you have problems.
- If you focus on life, you have life.
- If you focus on success, you will be successful.
- If you focus on the positive of everything, everything in your life will be positive.

A patient of mine asked me what the purpose of our life is, why we are in this world. I guess his suffering had brought on this kind of thought. I could not give an answer right away because everyone has a different answer. And I won't give you one, but I am interested in yours. So I leave this to you, my reader. You can send me e-mail, post through Facebook, or write me a postcard to discuss this question.

We need to raise awareness of our health, our bodies and minds, our lifestyles, our diets, and the best ways to get ourselves moving. We need to spread the word, telling people that there is a natural way for everything. We need to tell people, "Get up, move your body, and do something for your health." We need to open our minds and see things from a wider angle, not just from our usual narrow perspective. We need to accept what's true from both traditional science and nontraditional science. We need to pay attention to our own bodies, our own energy, our own issues, and our own behaviors, and stop putting the blame for our problems on others. We need to continue exploring, discovering, exercising, and, of course, never stop learning.

I wish you a great journey of exploring and learning.

Appendix: Remember the Dao

Below, I have included a few verses from the *Dao De Jing*, by the ancient Chinese philosopher Laozi. These excerpts come from *Backward Down the Path: A New Approach to the Tao Te Ching*, a fine translation by Jerry O. Dalton. The book was published by Humanics New Age.

63:3

> Deal with difficult things with simple acts.
>
> Deal with big things while they are small.
>
> Difficult tasks have easy beginnings.
>
> Large undertakings begin as small actions.

76:1

> At birth, a man is weak and flexible.
>
> At death, he is hard and rigid.
>
> All living things such as grass and trees,
>
> Are supple and yielding while alive,
>
> And withered and dry when they die.
>
> Thus unyielding rigidity is the companion of death,
>
> And yielding flexibility is the companion of life.

76:2

> Therefore an inflexible army will lose,
>
> The most rigid tree will snap.
>
> The hard and unyielding are lowered,
>
> While the soft and supple are elevated.

81:1

Truthful words are not beautiful,

Beautiful words are not true.

The wise man is not learned,

The learned man is not wise.

The good are not many,

The many are not good.

81:2

The sage does not accumulate things.

The more he does for others, the more he has.

The more he gives to others, the more he receives.

81:3

The Dao of heaven is to benefit without doing harm.

The Dao of the sage is to act without contending.

67.2

I have three treasures which I cherish and keep;

The first is compassion,

The second is frugality,

The third is not daring to go first in the world.

With compassion, one can be courageous.

With frugality, one can be generous.

With humility, one can be a leader of those who complete things.

If one is courageous without compassion,

If one is generous without frugality,

If one takes the lead without humility,

Then death is sure to follow.

Recommended Reading

Dalton, Jerry O. *Backward Down the Path: A New Approach to the Tao Te Ching*. Atlanta: Humanics New Age, 1994.

Dennison, Paul E., and Gail E. Dennison. *Brain Gym and Me*. Ventura, CA: Edu-Kinesthetics, Inc., 2006. (Please visit http://www.braingym.org.)

Dyer, Wayne W. *Change Your Thoughts—Change Your Life: Living the Wisdom of the Tao*. Carlsbad, CA: Hay House, 2007.

Formosa, Pamela. *Fraid Not: Empowering Kids with Learning Differences*. Bloomington, IN: iUniverse, 2009.

Frantzis, Bruce. *Tai Chi: Health for Life*. Berkeley, CA: Blue Snake Books, 2006.

Katz, Lawrence C., and Manning Rubins. *Keep Your Brain Alive: 83 Neurobic Exercises*. New York: Workman Publishing, 1998.

Kuhn, Aihan. *Natural Healing with Qigong: Therapeutic Qigong*. Boston: YMAA Publication Center, 2004.

———. *Simple Chinese Medicine: A Beginner's Guide to Natural Healing and Well-Being*. Boston, MA: YMAA Publication Center, 2009.

———. *Qi Gong for Travelers: Enhance Vitality Using Travel Time*. CreateSpace, 2013.

MacDonald, Matthew. *Your Brain: The Missing Manual*. Sebastopol, CA: Pogue Press, 2008.

Ratey, John J. *A User's Guide to the Brain*. New York: Random House, 2002.

Wing, R. L., trans. *The Tao of Power: Lao Tzu's Classic Guide to Leadership, Influence, and Excellence*. New York: Doubleday, 1986.

Yang, Jwing-Ming. *The Root of Chinese Qigong: Secrets for Health, Longevity, and Enlightenment*. Boston, MA: YMAA Publication Center, 1997.

Testimonials

Dr. Aihan Kuhn has once again shared with us a body of knowledge that can profoundly improve lives. She took a step beyond the neurological researchers who currently tell us what to expect as our brain ages. With her book, *Brain Fitness*, she gave us a road map for the path to the prevention of brain aging. This work is a valuable resource for both health-care practitioners and the individual who wants optimal health.

—Carl A.

As the population of the United States ages and the cost of health care sky rockets, alternative methods of healing are becoming very important. Dr. Kuhn's book *Brain Fitness* is a wonderful mix of Eastern and Western philosophy to help address some of these issues. With twenty-eight years of experience in the healing and martial arts, she has crafted a unique approach using taiji and qigong to keep the brain fit and healthy. The techniques found in her book are a must for anyone who wants to take control of their physical and mental health.

—Joe F.

Index

self-assessment, 84, 135

senior citizens, xii, 13, 15

shen, ii, xii, 11–12, 45, 75

shingles, 20

Simple Chinese Medicine (Kuhn), i, ii, iii, iv, v, vi, x, xi, xv, 14, 23, 56, 143, 145, 147–149

singing, ii, 53

sleep, 38–40

social activity, 50

soul, 12, 48

spirit, i, vi, xii, 10–12, 14–15, 45, 48, 50, 59, 63, 67–68, 75, 125, 134

stamina, i, 12, 20–21, 46, 53

stress, vi, 3, 5, 9, 12, 16–17, 22, 34, 44, 46–48, 54, 60, 66–68, 77, 84, 114, 134–136, 147–148

sympathetic nervous system (SNS), 19, 44

tai chi (*see* taiji), i, iv, vi, viii, 13, 20, 46, 84, 143, 147–149

Tai Chi for Depression (Kuhn), i, ii, iii, iv, v, vi, x, xi, xv, 13, 46, 56, 143, 145, 147–149

taiji, i, ii, vi, viii, x, xi, xii, xiii, xiv, xv, 2, 5–6, 8–24, 26–27, 30, 36–51, 57–59, 63, 65, 75–85, 104, 106, 129, 134, 145, 147

basics of

brain aging and, vi, xii, 14, 34, 46, 54

as brain exercise, 115

compared with qigong

described, vi, 80–81, 84–85

emotional benefits of

healing ability of

learning ability and, 46

as martial art

mental benefits of

movement requirements of

old school vs. new school

as perfect exercise

physical benefits of

practice requirements of

principles of, xiii, 75

qigong sequence

senior citizens and

sixteen-step form

spiritual benefits of

styles of, 57

Tao (*see* Dao), ii, 15, 62, 71, 141, 143

Tao of Power, The (Wing), 62, 71, 143

Tao Te Ching (*see* Dao De Jing), ii, 15, 141, 143

TCM (Traditional Chinese Medicine), ii, 12, 45, 54, 121, 147

television, 4, 42

thought processes, 37, 49, 62

thyroid, 22

touch, 49, 55, 62, 94, 96, 106, 108

traveling, 31, 62

trust, 66

tui na, 55, 148

vacationing, 31

values, 32

walking, 9–11, 15, 27, 51, 58, 63, 81, 85, 125

Wing, R. L., 62, 70–71, 143

yin and yang, 14–15, 30, 39, 77, 79, 105

Zhuang Z, 70i

About the Author

Dr. Aihan Kuhn is a unique doctor of natural medicine (holistic medicine). She is a speaker, an award-winning author, and a master of taiji and qigong. Trained in both conventional medicine and traditional Chinese medicine, Dr. Kuhn has helped thousands of patients overcome various physical ailments and emotional imbalances. She incorporates taiji and qigong into her healing methodologies, changing the lives of people who had struggled for many years and had no relief from conventional medicine. From her healing, patients also learn self-care techniques and strategies that help them to 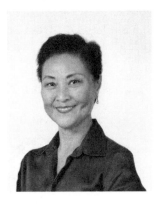 continue their healing journey at home. These techniques help self-confidence, relationships, stress management, daily energy level, and focus.

Dr. Kuhn provides many wellness programs, natural healing workshops, and professional training programs, such as her Tai Chi Instructor Training certification course, Qi Gong Instructor Training certification course, and Wellness Tui Na Therapy certification course. These highly rated programs have produced many quality teachers and therapists.

Dr. Kuhn is president of the Tai Chi & Qi Gong Healing Institute (www.TaiChi Healing.org), which is a nonprofit organization that promotes natural healing and prevention through an annual natural healing conference, World Tai Chi Day, healing qigong exercises, Daoist study, and special programs.

Dr. Kuhn now lives in Sarasota, Florida. She continues her natural healing education and offers consultations and private healing retreats for people who live far away to help them restore their health, inner balance, and vitality. For more information, please visit her website, www.draihankuhn.com.

Dr. Kuhn offers wellness education programs to help people improve their health, career, and overall quality of life. These programs include:

- The Secrets to Women's Health and Healing
- Natural Methods for Relief from Anxiety
- The Road to Fearless Living
- Relieve Stress in Seven Minutes
- Medicine, East Meets West
- Lose Weight in Seven Days
- Cancer Healing the Natural Way
- Weight Loss the Natural Way
- Qi Gong for Your Brain
- Emotion Healing through Body Movements
- Brain Fitness
- Food and Healing

Professional Training Programs (all of them offer continuing education credits for massage therapists):

- Qi Gong Instructor Training
- Tai Chi Instructor Training
- Wellness Tui Na Therapy
- Tui Na for Treating Common Ailments
- Tui Na for Back Therapy
- Tui Na for Neck Therapy

To find out more,
please visit:
www.DrAihanKuhn.com
www.taichihealing.org

Books by Dr. Kuhn:
Brain Fitness
Simple Chinese Medicine
Natural Healing with Qigong
Tai Chi for Depression
Weight Loss the Natural Way
Qigong for Travelers

Videos by Dr. Kuhn:
Tai Chi Chuan (24 Steps, Yang Style)
Tai Chi Chuan (42 Steps, Combined Style)
Tai Chi Chuan (24 Steps, Chen Style)
Tai Chi Sword (42 Steps, Combined Style)
Tai Chi Fan (Single Fan)
Tai Chi 16 Steps (for Internal Healing)
Therapeutic Qi Gong (36 Movements)
Meridian Qi Gong
Qi Gong for Arthritis
Circle Energy Qi Gong
Eight Brocade Qi Gong
Twelve Minutes Qi Gong for Computer Users
Tai Chi for Depression
Dr. Kuhn Tai Chi Form Collection

6 HEALING MOVEMENTS
101 REFLECTIONS ON TAI CHI CHUAN
108 INSIGHTS INTO TAI CHI CHUAN
ADVANCING IN TAE KWON DO
ANALYSIS OF SHAOLIN CHIN NA 2ND ED
ANCIENT CHINESE WEAPONS
THE ART AND SCIENCE OF STAFF FIGHTING
ART OF HOJO UNDO
ARTHRITIS RELIEF, 3D ED.
BACK PAIN RELIEF, 2ND ED.
BAGUAZHANG, 2ND ED.
BRAIN FITNESS
CARDIO KICKBOXING ELITE
CHIN NA IN GROUND FIGHTING
CHINESE FAST WRESTLING
CHINESE FITNESS
CHINESE TUI NA MASSAGE
CHOJUN
COMPREHENSIVE APPLICATIONS OF SHAOLIN CHIN NA
CONFLICT COMMUNICATION
CROCODILE AND THE CRANE: A NOVEL
CUTTING SEASON: A XENON PEARL MARTIAL ARTS THRILLER
DEFENSIVE TACTICS
DESHI: A CONNOR BURKE MARTIAL ARTS THRILLER
DIRTY GROUND
DR. WU'S HEAD MASSAGE
DUKKHA HUNGRY GHOSTS
DUKKHA REVERB
DUKKHA, THE SUFFERING: AN EYE FOR AN EYE
DUKKHA UNLOADED
ENZAN: THE FAR MOUNTAIN, A CONNOR BURKE MARTIAL
    ARTS THRILLER
ESSENCE OF SHAOLIN WHITE CRANE
EXPLORING TAI CHI
FACING VIOLENCE
FIGHT BACK
FIGHT LIKE A PHYSICIST
THE FIGHTER'S BODY
FIGHTER'S FACT BOOK
FIGHTER'S FACT BOOK 2
FIGHTING THE PAIN RESISTANT ATTACKER
FIRST DEFENSE
FORCE DECISIONS: A CITIZENS GUIDE
FOX BORROWS THE TIGER'S AWE
INSIDE TAI CHI
KAGE: THE SHADOW, A CONNOR BURKE MARTIAL ARTS
    THRILLER
KATA AND THE TRANSMISSION OF KNOWLEDGE
KRAV MAGA PROFESSIONAL TACTICS
KRAV MAGA WEAPON DEFENSES
LITTLE BLACK BOOK OF VIOLENCE
LIUHEBAFA FIVE CHARACTER SECRETS
MARTIAL ARTS ATHLETE
MARTIAL ARTS INSTRUCTION
MARTIAL WAY AND ITS VIRTUES
MASK OF THE KING
MEDITATIONS ON VIOLENCE
MERIDIAN QIGONG EXERCISES
MIND/BODY FITNESS
THE MIND INSIDE TAI CHI
THE MIND INSIDE YANG STYLE TAI CHI CHUAN
MUGAI RYU
NATURAL HEALING WITH QIGONG
NORTHERN SHAOLIN SWORD, 2ND ED.
OKINAWA'S COMPLETE KARATE SYSTEM: ISSHIN RYU
POWER BODY
PRINCIPLES OF TRADITIONAL CHINESE MEDICINE
QIGONG FOR HEALTH & MARTIAL ARTS 2ND ED.

QIGONG FOR LIVING
QIGONG FOR TREATING COMMON AILMENTS
QIGONG MASSAGE
QIGONG MEDITATION: EMBRYONIC BREATHING
QIGONG MEDITATION: SMALL CIRCULATION
QIGONG, THE SECRET OF YOUTH: DA MO'S CLASSICS
QUIET TEACHER: A XENON PEARL MARTIAL ARTS THRILLER
RAVEN'S WARRIOR
REDEMPTION
ROOT OF CHINESE QIGONG, 2ND ED.
SCALING FORCE
SENSEI: A CONNOR BURKE MARTIAL ARTS THRILLER
SHIHAN TE: THE BUNKAI OF KATA
SHIN GI TAI: KARATE TRAINING FOR BODY, MIND, AND SPIRIT
SIMPLE CHINESE MEDICINE
SIMPLE QIGONG EXERCISES FOR HEALTH, 3RD ED.
SIMPLIFIED TAI CHI CHUAN, 2ND ED.
SIMPLIFIED TAI CHI FOR BEGINNERS
SOLO TRAINING
SOLO TRAINING 2
SUDDEN DAWN: THE EPIC JOURNEY OF BODHIDHARMA
SUMO FOR MIXED MARTIAL ARTS
SUNRISE TAI CHI
SUNSET TAI CHI
SURVIVING ARMED ASSAULTS
TAE KWON DO: THE KOREAN MARTIAL ART
TAEKWONDO BLACK BELT POOMSAE
TAEKWONDO: A PATH TO EXCELLENCE
TAEKWONDO: ANCIENT WISDOM FOR THE MODERN
    WARRIOR
TAEKWONDO: DEFENSES AGAINST WEAPONS
TAEKWONDO: SPIRIT AND PRACTICE
TAO OF BIOENERGETICS
TAI CHI BALL QIGONG: FOR HEALTH AND MARTIAL ARTS
TAI CHI BALL WORKOUT FOR BEGINNERS
TAI CHI BOOK
TAI CHI CHIN NA: THE SEIZING ART OF TAI CHI CHUAN, 2ND
    ED.
TAI CHI CHUAN CLASSICAL YANG STYLE, 2ND ED.
TAI CHI CHUAN MARTIAL APPLICATIONS
TAI CHI CHUAN MARTIAL POWER, 3RD ED.
TAI CHI CONNECTIONS
TAI CHI DYNAMICS
TAI CHI FOR DEPRESSION
TAI CHI IN 10 WEEKS
TAI CHI QIGONG, 3RD ED.
TAI CHI SECRETS OF THE ANCIENT MASTERS
TAI CHI SECRETS OF THE WU & LI STYLES
TAI CHI SECRETS OF THE WU STYLE
TAI CHI SECRETS OF THE YANG STYLE
TAI CHI SWORD: CLASSICAL YANG STYLE, 2ND ED.
TAI CHI SWORD FOR BEGINNERS
TAI CHI WALKING
TAIJIQUAN THEORY OF DR. YANG, JWING-MING
TENGU: THE MOUNTAIN GOBLIN, A CONNOR BURKE
    MARTIAL ARTS THRILLER
TIMING IN THE FIGHTING ARTS
TRADITIONAL CHINESE HEALTH SECRETS
TRADITIONAL TAEKWONDO
TRAINING FOR SUDDEN VIOLENCE
WAY OF KATA
WAY OF KENDO AND KENJITSU
WAY OF SANCHIN KATA
WAY TO BLACK BELT
WESTERN HERBS FOR MARTIAL ARTISTS
WILD GOOSE QIGONG
WOMAN'S QIGONG GUIDE
XINGYIQUAN

DVDS FROM YMAA

more products available from . . .
YMAA Publication Center, Inc. 楊氏東方文化出版中心
1-800-669-8892 • info@ymaa.com • www.ymaa.com